Gastroenterology for

Beginners

Breaking Down Complex GI Medical Terminology and Vocabulary for High School / College Students and Patients

(Medical Terms Made Clear Series)

By **Richard J. Brooks**

Copyright Page

Gastroenterology for Beginners: Breaking Down Complex GI Medical Terminology and Vocabulary for High School / College Students and Patients

Disclaimer: This book is intended for **informational and educational** purposes only. It is **not** a substitute for professional medical advice, diagnosis, or treatment. Always seek the advice of qualified healthcare professionals with any questions you may have concerning a medical condition or procedure. The author and publisher assume **no liability** for any outcomes arising from the use of information contained herein.

Table of Contents

Chapter 1: Welcome to Gastroenterology 8

Chapter 2: Anatomy & Physiology of the GI Tract 18

Chapter 3: Common Diagnostic Tests & Procedures 29

Chapter 4: Upper GI Disorders—Esophagus & Stomach 40

Chapter 5: Small Intestine & Malabsorption Syndromes.........52

Chapter 6: Inflammatory Bowel Disease (IBD) — Crohn's &
Ulcerative Colitis 64

Chapter 7: Irritable Bowel Syndrome (IBS) & Functional
Disorders 75

Chapter 8: Colorectal Diseases & Screening 86

Chapter 9: Hepatology — Liver & Biliary Disorders 98

Chapter 10: Pancreatic Conditions.....................................111

Chapter 11: GI Infections & Parasites 121

Chapter 12: Pediatric Gastroenterology Essentials 131

Chapter 13: Lifestyle & Preventive Strategies 141

Chapter 14: FAQs & Common Myths in Gastroenterology ...151

Chapter 15: Glossary & Additional Resources 161

Dedication

To every individual striving to understand digestive health—may this book empower you to make more informed decisions about your well-being.

Acknowledgments

I wish to thank:

- **My esteemed gastroenterology colleagues**, who generously offered their insights and experiences to ensure accuracy.
- **Friends and family**, for their continuous support and patience throughout the writing process.
- **Readers**, whose questions about the GI tract inspired a clearer, friendlier approach to medical terminology.

Foreword

Foreword by Dr. Nicole Abeli, MD (Gastroenterologist)

The GI system plays a foundational role in nourishment and overall health, yet it's often cloaked in complex terms. In *Gastroenterology for Beginners*, Richard J. Brooks transforms these concepts into accessible lessons that both new learners and patients will find enlightening. By blending concise definitions with this book demystifies everything from acid reflux to inflammatory bowel disease—an essential guide for anyone aiming to better understand digestive processes and disorders.

Preface

Why This Book?

Digestion is both straightforward—turning food into energy—and astonishingly complex, involving multiple organs, enzymes, and an ecosystem of microbes. Yet, conversations about the GI tract frequently dissolve into unfamiliar abbreviations and technical jargon, which can discourage further inquiry.

In **Gastroenterology for Beginners**, I've aimed to **simplify** the language without sacrificing **accuracy**, giving you the tools to navigate topics like GI anatomy, common disorders, diagnostic tests, and cutting-edge treatments. Whether you're a **student**, **patient**, or simply curious about digestive health, you'll find approachable explanations and practical insights here.

Who Will Benefit?

- **High School or College Students** preparing for exams or exploring healthcare careers.
- **Patients & Caregivers** wanting clear definitions of terms often mentioned in endoscopy reports or medical consultations.
- **General Enthusiasts** who wish to appreciate how their body processes nutrients and signals distress.

How to Use This Book

- **Chapter-by-Chapter Learning**: Each section covers a key aspect of gastroenterology—anatomy, disease states, interventions—ending with a "Key Terms Recap & Quiz."
- **Glossary**: At the end for quick cross-referencing terms or finding specific topics.
- **Additional Resources**: Pointers to reputable websites, support groups, and professional organizations for deeper exploration.

With these chapters, I hope to strip away intimidation, fostering **confidence** in understanding your GI system or caring for those with digestive concerns. Let's begin the journey into the intricate world of digestion and gut health.

Chapter 1: Welcome to Gastroenterology

1.1 Why the GI Tract Matters

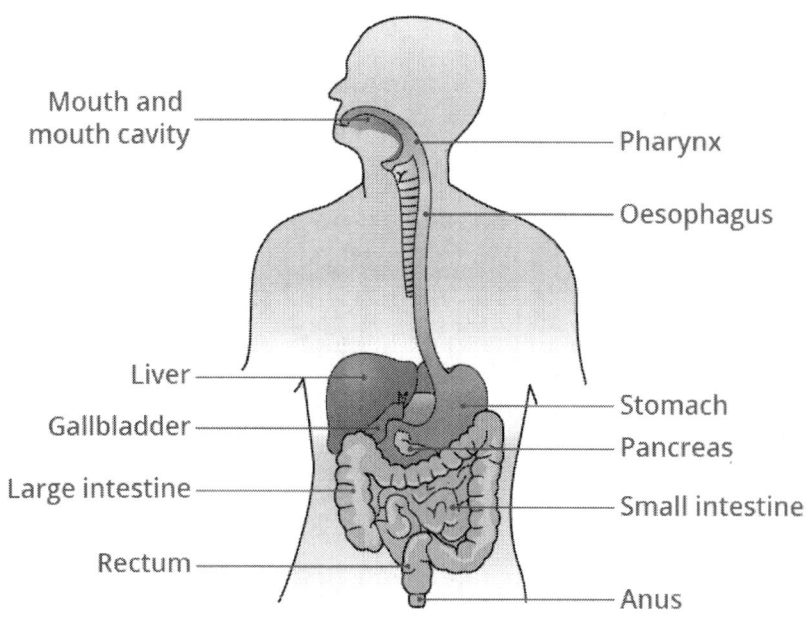

The gastrointestinal (GI) tract is often described as a **food-processing factory**, but it's far more than just an assembly line for digestion. A healthy GI system underpins our **nutritional status**, shapes our **immune responses**, and even influences our **hormonal balance** and mood via the gut-brain axis. Let's break down why the GI tract is so crucial.

1.1.1 Digestive Processes & Nutrient Absorption

- **Mouth to Intestines**: The journey of food begins with chewing, mixing with saliva, and swallowing. Once in the stomach and small intestine, powerful enzymes and acids break down proteins, fats, and carbohydrates.
- **Absorption**: The small intestine, lined with **villi** and **microvilli**, provides an enormous surface area for nutrients, vitamins, and minerals to cross into the bloodstream. A failure at this step (such as in **celiac disease** or **short bowel syndrome**) leads to malabsorption, malnutrition, and systemic deficits.
- **Metabolism**: The liver, pancreas, and gallbladder produce or store essential substances (bile, enzymes, hormones) that further optimize digestion and assimilation of nutrients.

1.1.2 Immune Function & Microbiome

- **GI Lining**: A large part of the body's immune system resides in the gut-associated lymphoid tissue (GALT), capable of defending against ingested pathogens.
- **Microbiome**: Trillions of microbes inhabit our intestines. These bacteria, viruses, and fungi help ferment dietary

fibers, synthesize certain vitamins, and regulate immune responses. Disruptions (dysbiosis) can contribute to conditions like inflammatory bowel disease (IBD) or irritable bowel syndrome (IBS).

- **Protective Barrier**: A healthy gut lining prevents harmful substances from entering the bloodstream, supporting the concept of "leaky gut" when damaged or inflamed.

1.1.3 Overall Health Implications

A malfunction in any segment of the GI system can ripple through the entire body. Chronic digestive disorders (e.g., **GERD, Crohn's disease, non-alcoholic fatty liver disease**) can reduce quality of life, lead to nutrient deficiencies, or predispose to life-threatening complications like **colon cancer** or **cirrhosis**. Understanding GI terms and disease processes is thus essential for robust health management.

1.2 Who This Book Is For

1.2.1 High School/College Students & New Healthcare Learners

If you're a **student** exploring biology or considering a healthcare career (nursing, pre-med, allied health), you'll find:

- **Plain-Language Explanations**: Simplified definitions of complex GI terms like "peristalsis," "fistula," or "transaminases."
- **Recap Quizzes**: Reinforcing knowledge after each chapter.

1.2.2 Patients & Caregivers With GI Concerns

Navigating the medical system with a **digestive diagnosis** (GERD, IBS, hepatitis, etc.) can be overwhelming. This book helps by:

- **Decoding Medical Jargon**: Understand your endoscopy report, lab results, or biopsy findings.
- **Answering FAQs**: Common worries like "Is this procedure painful?" "What does this test mean for me?"
- **Treatment Overviews**: Awareness of standard therapies (medications, lifestyle changes) and potential surgical options.

1.2.3 General Readers Curious About Digestive Health

Even if you have no immediate GI issue, you might be fascinated by how the body turns food into energy and discards waste. By reading these chapters, you'll get:

- **Insight Into Preventive Strategies**: Diet, exercise, and screening that lower the risk of GI problems.
- **Better Grasp of Nutrition**: Understand fiber, vitamins, and how gut microbes influence well-being.
- **Confidence** in reading about or discussing GI topics (like the latest probiotics or colon cancer screening guidelines).

1.3 Structure & Key Features

Gastroenterology for Beginners follows a **consistent format** to keep learning streamlined and enjoyable:

1. **Chapter Objectives**: Each chapter starts with a clear statement of what you'll learn—whether it's understanding how the stomach processes food or exploring how colonoscopy detects polyps.
2. **Core Content**: Key definitions, pathophysiology, common tests, and therapies. We emphasize everyday language, ensuring technical terms are introduced with user-friendly explanations.
3. **Key Terms Recap & Quiz**: A short bullet list highlighting vital terms from the chapter, followed by multiple-choice or short-answer questions to reinforce memory and comprehension.

1.3.1 Glossary

- **Glossary**: Located at the end of the book, providing succinct definitions for over 100 GI terms, from "achalasia" to "Zollinger-Ellison syndrome."

1.3.2 Additional Resources & References

In the closing pages, you'll find:

- **Professional Organizations**: (American College of Gastroenterology, AGA) for advanced guidelines.
- **Support Groups**: IBS, IBD, celiac disease foundations.
- **Online Educational Sites**: Verified medical resources for deeper reading.

1.4 Chapter Summaries: A Preview

Below is a quick **snapshot** of what the upcoming chapters will cover:

1. **Anatomy & Physiology of the GI Tract** (Chapter 2)
   - Detailed walkthrough from mouth to colon, plus accessory organs (liver, pancreas).
   - Essential for grasping how digestion, absorption, and gut motility function together.
2. **Common Diagnostic Tests & Procedures** (Chapter 3)

- Endoscopies, imaging techniques (CT/MRI), lab analyses (stool, breath tests).
- How these tests pinpoint issues like ulcers, tumors, or malabsorption.

3. **Upper GI Disorders: Esophagus & Stomach** (Chapter 4)
- GERD, peptic ulcers, gastritis. Key terms like *H. pylori*, PPIs, acid reflux.
- Understanding alarm symptoms and when to see a specialist.

4. **Small Intestine & Malabsorption Syndromes** (Chapter 5)
- Celiac disease, tropical sprue, short bowel syndrome.
- Nutritional consequences and management strategies.

5. **Inflammatory Bowel Disease (IBD): Crohn's & Ulcerative Colitis** (Chapter 6)
- Comparing features, complications, modern treatments (immunomodulators, biologics).

6. **Irritable Bowel Syndrome (IBS) & Functional Disorders** (Chapter 7)
- Rome IV criteria, stress-related triggers, dietary management.
- Clarifying differences between functional GI issues and structural diseases.

7. **Colorectal Diseases & Screening** (Chapter 8)
   ○ Polyps, colorectal cancer, diverticular disease.
   ○ Importance of colonoscopy and polypectomy in prevention.
8. **Hepatology: Liver & Biliary Disorders** (Chapter 9)
   ○ Viral hepatitis, cirrhosis, cholelithiasis.
   ○ Key labs (LFTs), imaging (MRCP).
9. **Pancreatic Conditions** (Chapter 10)
   ○ Acute vs. chronic pancreatitis, pancreatic cancer, enzyme replacement therapy.
10. **GI Infections & Parasites** (Chapter 11)
    ○ Common bacterial, viral, parasitic pathogens.
    ○ Supportive vs. targeted antimicrobial treatments.
11. **Pediatric Gastroenterology Essentials** (Chapter 12)
    ○ Reflux in infants, common malabsorption (milk protein allergy), toddler constipation.
    ○ Unique pediatric GI physiology.
12. **Lifestyle & Preventive Strategies** (Chapter 13)
    ○ Diet, exercise, screening tests, immunizations, stress management.
    ○ Maintaining healthy digestion through proactive habits.
13. **FAQs & Common Myths in Gastroenterology** (Chapter 14)

- Dispelling misconceptions: "Spicy food always causes ulcers," "You don't need screenings if you have no symptoms," etc.
- Quick tips on second opinions, medication adherence.

14. **Glossary & Additional Resources** (Chapter 15)
    - A final reference to key terminology and recommended reading.

With each chapter, you'll see **consistent structure**, **straightforward language**, and a **practical approach** to understanding digestive health, ensuring you're armed with the knowledge to interpret GI tests, manage chronic conditions, or just improve everyday digestive wellness.

1.5 Final Thoughts on Chapter 1

This **introductory chapter** sets the stage for a clear, cohesive journey into gastrointestinal medicine. The GI system is fundamental to energy production, immunity, and overall vitality. By exploring **how** it works and **what** goes wrong in common diseases, you'll develop a more empowered viewpoint—be it as a student, healthcare aspirant, patient, or curious reader.

In **Chapter 2**, we begin with a **deep dive into GI Anatomy & Physiology**, examining each major organ from the mouth to the intestines, plus the supportive roles of the liver, gallbladder, and pancreas. Understanding the normal architecture and function is critical before dissecting pathologies like reflux, IBS, or liver cirrhosis. Get ready to uncover the fascinating intricacies of digestion, absorption, and the unseen world inside your gut!

Key Points Recap

- **GI System Importance**: Manages digestion, nutrient absorption, immune defense.
- **Who Benefits**: Students, patients, general health enthusiasts wanting to decode GI terms.
- **Book Structure**: Chapters feature clear objectives, quizzes, and a glossary for quick reference.
- **Next Step**: **Chapter 2**—a thorough exploration of **GI anatomy and physiology**, providing the backbone for understanding diseases and their management.

Chapter 2: Anatomy & Physiology of the GI Tract

2.1 Mouth & Esophagus

2.1.1 Chewing & Salivary Enzymes

Digestion starts in the **mouth**, where **mechanical** and **chemical** processes begin:

1. **Mastication (Chewing)**
   - Teeth grind solid food into smaller pieces, increasing its surface area for enzyme action.
   - The tongue helps reposition food for efficient chewing, then forms a **bolus** ready to swallow.
2. **Salivary Glands & Enzymes**
   - **Saliva** contains water, mucus, electrolytes, and enzymes (like **amylase**, which begins starch breakdown, and **lingual lipase**, which acts on fats especially in infants).
   - Saliva moistens food, making swallowing smoother, and has some antimicrobial properties (lysozymes, IgA).
3. **Taste & Pleasure**

- Papillae on the tongue sense sweet, sour, salty, bitter, and umami, prompting saliva production.
- Enjoyment of flavors can stimulate further digestive secretions throughout the GI tract.

2.1.2 Swallowing Mechanics

Swallowing (deglutition) involves coordinated muscle contractions and reflexes:

1. **Oral Phase**
   - Voluntary portion: The tongue pushes the bolus to the back of the mouth toward the oropharynx.
2. **Pharyngeal Phase**
   - Involuntary reflex seals off the nasopharynx (soft palate elevates) and blocks the airway with the **epiglottis**.
   - Bolus passes the upper esophageal sphincter into the esophagus.
3. **Esophageal Phase**
   - **Peristalsis** (rhythmic, wave-like muscle contractions) propels the bolus downward.
   - The **lower esophageal sphincter (LES)** relaxes to allow entry into the stomach, then closes to prevent reflux of acidic contents.

2.2 Stomach

2.2.1 Acid Secretion & Pepsin

The stomach's environment is uniquely acidic, thanks to parietal cells secreting **hydrochloric acid (HCl)**:

1. **Parietal Cells**
   - Pump H^+ ions into the lumen, achieving a highly **acidic pH (~1–3)**.
   - Intrinsic factor secretion is crucial for vitamin B_{12} absorption later in the ileum.
2. **Chief Cells**
   - Produce **pepsinogen**, which HCl activates to **pepsin**, an enzyme that begins protein digestion.
3. **Mucus Cells**
   - Mucus and bicarbonate form a protective layer against self-digestion by acid.
   - Disruption of this barrier can lead to peptic ulcers.

2.2.2 Mechanical Churning & Terms

The stomach also **mixes** and churns the bolus with gastric secretions, creating **chyme**—a semi-liquid mixture. Key terms:

- **Rugae**: Folds in the stomach lining that stretch as the stomach fills.
- **Chyme**: The acidic slurry that moves into the duodenum.

- **pH**: In the stomach, typically very low (acidic). Regulatory hormones (gastrin, secretin) help moderate acid production.

2.3 Small Intestine

2.3.1 Duodenum, Jejunum, Ileum

The **small intestine** is the primary site for digestion and absorption. Its sections each have specialized roles:

1. **Duodenum**
   - Receives **chyme** from the stomach plus **bile** (from the liver/gallbladder) and **pancreatic enzymes** (lipase, amylase, proteases).
   - Neutralizes stomach acid via bicarbonate secretions.
2. **Jejunum**
   - Major site of nutrient absorption. Highly vascularized, with prominent **villi** to maximize surface area.
3. **Ileum**
   - Continues absorption (especially vitamin B_{12} and bile salts).
   - Ends at the ileocecal valve, controlling flow into the large intestine.

2.3.2 Enzymes & Nutrient Absorption

1. **Brush Border Enzymes**
   - Located on microvilli, finalizing the breakdown of carbohydrates (disaccharidases like lactase, sucrase) and proteins (peptidases).
   - Deficiency (e.g., lactase deficiency) leads to malabsorption and intolerance.

2. **Villous Structure**
   - **Villi**: Finger-like projections lined by enterocytes.
   - **Microvilli**: Tiny projections on each cell, forming the "brush border."
   - This design **massively expands** the surface area, crucial for efficient absorption of amino acids, monosaccharides, fats (packaged into chylomicrons), vitamins, and minerals.

3. **Motility**:
   - **Peristalsis** and **segmentation** move chyme along and ensure thorough mixing with enzymes.

2.4 Large Intestine

2.4.1 Water Reabsorption & Fecal Formation

After the small intestine absorbs most nutrients, the **large intestine** (colon) focuses on:

1. **Water & Electrolyte Reabsorption**
   - The colon recovers fluid, converting liquid chyme into more solid stool.
   - Disturbances (like infection or inflammation) can lead to diarrhea or constipation.
2. **Gut Microbiome**
   - Trillions of bacteria assist in fermenting residual fibers, producing short-chain fatty acids beneficial for colon health.
   - Disruptions in microbiome composition can influence conditions like IBS, IBD, or obesity.
3. **Stool Formation & Storage**
   - Indigestible remnants, bacterial mass, and sloughed cells form feces.
   - Stored in the rectum until defecation reflex triggers elimination.

2.4.2 Segments & Functions

- **Cecum & Appendix**: Junction with the ileum; the appendix may have immunological roles.
- **Ascending, Transverse, Descending, Sigmoid Colon**: Progressive absorption, fecal compaction.
- **Rectum & Anus**: Final storage and controlled passage (internal/external sphincters).

2.5 Accessory Organs: Liver, Gallbladder, Pancreas

2.5.1 Liver

One of the body's metabolic powerhouses, the **liver**:

1. **Produces Bile**
   - Bile salts emulsify fats, aiding fat digestion. Also a route for bilirubin and cholesterol excretion.
2. **Metabolizes Nutrients**
   - Processes glucose (glycogen storage), amino acids, lipids.
3. **Detoxification**
   - Inactivates or excretes drugs, toxins, hormones.
4. **Protein Synthesis**
   - Albumin for oncotic pressure, clotting factors (coagulation).

2.5.2 Gallbladder

- **Bile Storage & Concentration**
   - Contracts post-meal to release bile into the duodenum via the common bile duct.

- Gallstones form if bile components (cholesterol, bilirubin) crystallize, potentially causing biliary colic or cholecystitis.

2.5.3 Pancreas

Two major functions:

1. **Exocrine**
   - Secretes digestive enzymes (amylase for carbs, lipase for fats, proteases like trypsin) into the duodenum.
   - Bicarbonate solution buffers acidic chyme.
2. **Endocrine**
   - **Islets of Langerhans** produce insulin (lowers blood glucose) and glucagon (raises blood glucose).
   - Dysregulation leads to diabetes mellitus.

2.6 Key Terms: Peristalsis, Sphincters, Villi, Microvilli

- **Peristalsis**: Coordinated, wave-like muscle contractions propelling contents along the GI tract, from esophagus to rectum.

- **Sphincters**: Circular muscle "valves" that regulate flow between sections (e.g., lower esophageal sphincter, pyloric sphincter).
- **Villi**: Fingerlike projections in the small intestine increasing surface area for absorption.
- **Microvilli**: Tiny projections on each epithelial cell's apical surface, forming the "brush border" with embedded enzymes.

Understanding these four terms is foundational. Each highlights the GI tract's structural sophistication—coordinating muscular motion, segmented compartments, and a finely tuned surface for nutrient uptake.

2.7 Quick Quiz

Test your comprehension of GI **anatomy & physiology**:

1. **Multiple Choice**: Which organ primarily **neutralizes** acidic chyme from the stomach by secreting bicarbonate-rich fluid?
   a) Liver
   b) Pancreas
   c) Gallbladder
   d) Small intestine (Ileum)
2. **True or False**: **Peristalsis** is exclusively a stomach-based mechanism.

3. **Fill in the Blank**: The innermost surface of the small intestine is covered with tiny projections called _____, which are further lined by even smaller _____ to maximize absorption.

4. **Short Answer**: Why do we say the **liver** is a "metabolic powerhouse" in the body?

5. **Which GI segment is most responsible for absorbing water and consolidating waste into feces?**
   a) Duodenum
   b) Stomach
   c) Large intestine (Colon)
   d) Pancreas

Answers

1. **(b) Pancreas** – Releases bicarbonate into the duodenum to neutralize the acidic chyme.
2. **False** – Peristalsis occurs throughout the GI tract (esophagus, intestines, etc.).
3. **Villi, microvilli** – Key structural components for nutrient absorption in the small intestine.
4. **Example**: "Because it metabolizes nutrients (carbs, proteins, fats), detoxifies chemicals, produces bile, and synthesizes vital proteins and coagulation factors."

5. **(c) Large intestine** – Absorbs water/electrolytes, forms feces.

Concluding Note

From chewing in the **mouth** to final waste formation in the **colon**, the GI tract orchestrates a symphony of enzymes, muscular contractions, and specialized cells. **Sphincters** and **peristalsis** ensure one-way flow, while **villi** and **microvilli** optimize nutrient uptake. The **stomach** churns and acidifies, the **small intestine** performs the lion's share of absorption, and the **large intestine** recovers water and houses beneficial bacteria. Meanwhile, **accessory organs** like the liver, gallbladder, and pancreas provide crucial secretions—bile, enzymes, and hormones—that refine digestion and metabolism.

In **Chapter 3**, we'll examine the **Common Diagnostic Tests & Procedures** in gastroenterology—ranging from **endoscopic** exams (EGD, colonoscopy) to specialized imaging and stool studies—offering a blueprint for how doctors pinpoint and monitor GI disorders with remarkable precision.

Chapter 3: Common Diagnostic Tests & Procedures

3.1 Endoscopies

3.1.1 EGD (Esophagogastroduodenoscopy)

Esophagogastroduodenoscopy (EGD), sometimes called **upper endoscopy**, allows direct visualization of the **esophagus**, **stomach**, and **duodenum** via a thin, flexible scope:

1. **Purpose & Indications**
   - Investigate causes of **dyspepsia** (persistent indigestion), **GERD** complications, suspected **peptic ulcers**, or upper GI bleeding.
   - Obtain **biopsies** to check for H. pylori, celiac disease, or suspicious lesions.
2. **Procedure Overview**
   - Generally performed under sedation.
   - The endoscope has a camera and light; the doctor can inflate air for better visibility and use

tiny instruments for biopsies or to control bleeding.

3. **Key Benefits**
   - Direct inspection helps detect erosions, ulcers, tumors.
   - Therapeutic uses: removing polyps in the stomach, banding varices, treating bleeding ulcers with injection or cautery.

3.1.2 Colonoscopy

Colonoscopy focuses on the **colon** (large intestine) and distal ileum:

1. **Why It's Done**
   - Gold standard for **colon cancer screening**: can detect and remove polyps before they progress to malignancy.
   - Investigate chronic diarrhea, rectal bleeding, unexplained weight loss, or suspected inflammatory bowel disease.
2. **Preparation**
   - Bowel prep (laxatives, clear-liquid diet) essential for clear visualization.
   - Sedation often provided for patient comfort.
3. **Polypectomy & Biopsies**

- Polyps are snared off or biopsied to determine pathology (adenomatous vs. hyperplastic).
- Tissue samples confirm conditions like ulcerative colitis, Crohn's, or microscopic colitis.

3.1.3 Sigmoidoscopy

Sigmoidoscopy examines only the **distal part** of the colon (sigmoid and rectum). It can be:

- **Flexible Sigmoidoscopy**: Less extensive than a full colonoscopy, often no sedation needed.
- **Indications**: Quick assessment of rectal bleeding, distal colitis, or polyp follow-up.
- **Limitations**: Doesn't detect proximal colon issues that might be missed if pathology lies beyond the reach of the scope.

3.2 Imaging

3.2.1 Abdominal Ultrasound

Ultrasound uses sound waves to visualize soft tissues:

- **Liver & Gallbladder**: Checking for gallstones, biliary dilation, or hepatic lesions.

- **Pancreas**: Basic structural assessment if no overlying bowel gas interference.
- **Kidneys & Aorta**: Though not GI per se, often scanned in abdominal ultrasound.
- **Advantages**: No radiation, real-time scanning, low cost.

3.2.2 CT Scans

A **CT (Computed Tomography)** scan offers **cross-sectional** X-ray images for detailed GI organ views:

1. **Abdominal/Pelvic CT**
    - Identifies masses, inflammation, abscesses, or abnormal fluid collections.
    - Guides biopsy or intervention if needed.
2. **Contrast Enhancement**
    - Intravenous (IV) or oral contrast helps delineate blood vessels, differentiate tissues.
    - "CT Enterography" specialized for small bowel imaging.
3. **Radiation Considerations**
    - CT scans involve more radiation than ultrasound or MRI, thus used when benefits outweigh risks.

3.2.3 MRI (Including MRCP)

MRI (Magnetic Resonance Imaging) excels at soft tissue contrast without radiation:

- **MRCP (Magnetic Resonance Cholangiopancreatography)**
  - Specialized MRI sequence visualizing biliary and pancreatic ducts.
  - Non-invasive alternative to ERCP (endoscopic retrograde cholangiopancreatography) for detecting stones, strictures, or congenital anomalies.

3.2.4 Contrast Studies

- **Barium Swallow** (Esophagram)
  - Drinking barium highlights the esophageal lumen on X-ray, diagnosing strictures, motility disorders.
- **Barium Enema**
  - Outlines the colon, detecting masses or strictures if colonoscopy is incomplete or not feasible.
- **Limitations**: Less common nowadays, with endoscopy being more definitive, but still used in certain scenarios (like suspected advanced motility disorders).

3.3 Laboratory Workups

3.3.1 Stool Tests

1. **Occult Blood Test (FOBT, FIT)**
   - Screens for hidden blood in stool, aiding early detection of colon polyps or cancer.
2. **Stool Culture**
   - Identifies pathogens (bacteria, parasites) in infectious diarrhea.
3. **Fecal Calprotectin**
   - Marker of intestinal inflammation—differentiates IBD from irritable bowel syndrome (IBS).

3.3.2 Breath Tests

- **H. pylori Urea Breath Test**
  - Detects Helicobacter pylori, a common culprit in peptic ulcers.
- **Lactose Intolerance Test**
  - Measures hydrogen exhaled after consuming lactose; elevated in lactose malabsorption.

3.3.3 Other Labs

- **Serologic Markers**: Celiac serology (tTG-IgA), viral hepatitis panels.
- **Pancreatic Enzymes**: Amylase, lipase for suspected pancreatitis.

- **Liver Function Tests (LFTs)**: AST, ALT, alkaline phosphatase, bilirubin.

3.4 Esophageal pH Monitoring & Manometry

3.4.1 GERD Assessment

24-hour esophageal pH monitoring measures acid reflux episodes over a day:

- **Procedure**: A thin probe in the esophagus (or a wireless capsule attached to the esophageal lining) records pH.
- **Indications**: Atypical or refractory GERD symptoms, preoperative evaluation for fundoplication.

3.4.2 Manometry

Manometry evaluates **muscular contractions** and **pressures** within the esophagus or anorectal region:

1. **Esophageal Manometry**
   - Diagnoses motility disorders (achalasia, diffuse esophageal spasm).
   - Identifies abnormal peristalsis, LES dysfunction (weak or hypertensive sphincter).
2. **Anorectal Manometry**

- Assesses sphincter function for fecal incontinence or chronic constipation.

Note: These specialized tests clarify functional GI disorders when endoscopy or imaging appear normal.

3.5 Biopsy Techniques

3.5.1 Forceps Biopsy & Brush Cytology

During endoscopy:

1. **Forceps Biopsy**
   - Small jaw-like forceps pinch off tissue samples (e.g., from a suspicious ulcer, a polyp).
   - Histopathology reveals inflammation (gastritis, colitis) or malignancy.
2. **Brush Cytology**
   - A tiny brush collects surface cells for cytological study, helpful for esophageal strictures or suspicious lumps.
   - Less invasive but may yield smaller samples.

3.5.2 Polypectomy

Polypectomy is the removal of polyps (often in the colon) using a snare or cautery:

- **Diagnostic & Therapeutic**: Pathology identifies benign vs. malignant potential, removing the polyp can prevent cancer development.
- **Complications**: Rarely bleeding or perforation, typically minimal with careful technique.

3.6 Key Terms Recap

- **EGD (Esophagogastroduodenoscopy)**: Visual exam of the upper GI tract.
- **Colonoscopy**: Scope to inspect the colon, essential in colon cancer screening.
- **MRI/MRCP**: Magnetic resonance imaging for GI organs; MRCP targets bile/pancreatic ducts.
- **Manometry**: Evaluates motility and pressure within the esophagus or anal canal.
- **Polypectomy**: Snaring/removing polyps during colonoscopy to prevent progression to cancer.
- **Stool Tests (FOBT, FIT)**: Detect hidden blood or pathogens in feces.

3.7 Quick Quiz

1. **Multiple Choice**: Which test is often deemed the "gold standard" for diagnosing and removing colonic polyps?
   a) Barium enema

b) CT colonography

c) Colonoscopy

d) Stool occult blood test

2. **True or False**: An EGD can help identify gastritis or duodenal ulcers and obtain biopsies for H. pylori testing.

3. **Fill in the Blank**: _____ measures the acid level in the esophagus over 24 hours, aiding in diagnosing atypical or severe GERD.

4. **Which imaging method is especially useful for evaluating biliary and pancreatic ductal anatomy without needing an invasive endoscopic approach?**

a) ERCP

b) MRCP

c) Plain abdominal X-ray

d) Esophagram

5. **Short Answer**: Name one advantage of a flexible sigmoidoscopy over a colonoscopy, and one disadvantage.

Answers

1. **(c) Colonoscopy** – The definitive approach for polyp detection and removal.

2. **True** – EGD can visually confirm ulcers/gastritis and collect biopsy samples.

3. **24-hour esophageal pH monitoring** – Sometimes referred to as a "pH probe" study.
4. **(b) MRCP** – Non-invasive MRI sequence to visualize bile and pancreatic ducts.
5. **Example**: "Flexible sigmoidoscopy is quicker, often needs less sedation, but it only examines the distal colon and can miss proximal lesions."

Concluding Note

From **endoscopy** to **manometry**, **biopsy** to **imaging**, gastroenterology is rich in **diagnostic tools** allowing precise detection and management of a wide range of digestive conditions. Understanding each test's purpose, preparation, and scope clarifies why doctors may recommend them—and can help patients (or students) approach procedures with more confidence.

In **Chapter 4**, we'll zoom in on **Upper GI Disorders: Esophagus & Stomach**, looking at **GERD**, **peptic ulcer disease**, and related conditions. The knowledge of how these tests confirm or differentiate these disorders will become all the more relevant as we delve deeper into the specifics of GI pathologies.

Chapter 4: Upper GI Disorders—Esophagus & Stomach

4.1 GERD (Gastroesophageal Reflux Disease)

4.1.1 Pathophysiology

Gastroesophageal reflux disease (GERD) arises when **stomach acid** and sometimes bile reflux into the **esophagus**, causing irritation or even structural damage:

1. **Lower Esophageal Sphincter (LES) Dysfunction**
   - The LES normally prevents backflow from the stomach. In GERD, it's weakened or relaxes inappropriately, allowing acid to escape upward.
   - Contributors: high intra-abdominal pressure (obesity, pregnancy), hiatal hernia, certain foods (chocolate, mint), or medications (anticholinergics, calcium channel blockers).
2. **Acid-Induced Injury**

- The esophageal lining lacks the protective mucus-bicarbonate layer found in the stomach. Repeated acid contact → inflammation (esophagitis), erosions, ulcerations.

3. **Associated Factors**
   - **Transient LES Relaxations**: Part of normal swallowing, but can be too frequent.
   - **Lifestyle**: Large meals before lying down, fatty meals slowing gastric emptying, smoking weakening LES further.

4.1.2 Symptoms & Complications

1. **Common Symptoms**
   - **Heartburn** (burning sensation in the retrosternal area), often post-meal or when reclining.
   - **Regurgitation** of acid or food into the mouth.
   - Possible **chest pain** mimicking cardiac issues, sore throat, hoarseness (if reflux affects vocal cords).

2. **Alarm Features**
   - Dysphagia (trouble swallowing), odynophagia (painful swallowing).

- GI bleeding (dark stools, anemia) or significant weight loss.
- These may indicate complications like strictures or esophageal cancer.

3. **Barrett's Esophagus**
   - Chronic acid damage → **metaplastic change** of the lower esophageal lining, raising risk of adenocarcinoma (discussed more later in this chapter).

4.1.3 Management

1. **Lifestyle Modifications**
   - Weight reduction, elevating the head of the bed, avoiding trigger foods (spicy, acidic) and late-night meals, quitting smoking.
   - Smaller, more frequent meals to reduce gastric volume.
2. **Medications**
   - **PPIs (Proton Pump Inhibitors)**: Omeprazole, esomeprazole, etc. Potently reduce acid secretion, promote healing.
   - **H2 Blockers**: Ranitidine, famotidine; less potent but still effective for mild cases.
   - **Antacids & Alginates**: Quick symptomatic relief, neutralize acid or form a protective raft.

3. **Surgical Option**: Nissen Fundoplication
    - The gastric fundus is wrapped around the distal esophagus, reinforcing the LES barrier. Reserved for refractory cases or when long-term medication is poorly tolerated.

4.2 Peptic Ulcer Disease (PUD)

4.2.1 Helicobacter pylori & NSAIDs

Peptic ulcers are open sores in the **stomach** (gastric ulcers) or **duodenum** (duodenal ulcers). Two major causes:

1. **Helicobacter pylori (H. pylori)**
    - A spiral-shaped bacterium colonizing gastric mucosa.
    - Produces urease (neutralizing acid locally), causing chronic gastritis and, over time, ulcer formation.
    - Associated with gastric cancer and MALT lymphoma in some patients.
2. **NSAID Overuse**
    - Nonsteroidal anti-inflammatory drugs (ibuprofen, naproxen) inhibit prostaglandin production, reducing the protective mucus layer in the stomach/duodenum.

- This vulnerability to acid can result in mucosal erosions or deeper ulcers.

4.2.2 Gastric vs. Duodenal Ulcers

1. **Gastric Ulcers**
   - Often worsened by eating; patients might lose weight from fear of pain.
   - Greater risk of malignancy than duodenal ulcers—biopsy typically recommended.
2. **Duodenal Ulcers**
   - Classically, pain **relieved by food**, returning hours later when the stomach is empty.
   - More common overall, strongly linked to H. pylori infection.

4.2.3 Symptoms & Alarm Features

1. **Symptoms**
   - Epigastric pain (burning, gnawing), possible nocturnal flare-ups, sometimes relief with antacids.
   - If an ulcer erodes into a blood vessel, melena (black tarry stools) or hematemesis can occur.
2. **Alarm Features**

- Bleeding (anemia, black stools), perforation (sudden severe abdominal pain, peritonitis), obstruction (persistent vomiting).
- Urgent endoscopy to identify location and severity of ulcers.

4.2.4 Eradication Therapy for H. pylori

1. **Diagnosis:**
   - Urea breath test, stool antigen test, or biopsy-based tests (rapid urease test).
2. **Triple or Quadruple Therapy:**
   - **PPI + 2 antibiotics** (e.g., clarithromycin + amoxicillin) ± bismuth.
   - Duration typically 10–14 days; confirm eradication if ulcer complications or high risk of recurrence.
3. **NSAID Management**
   - If NSAIDs essential, add prophylactic PPI. Consider alternative analgesics (acetaminophen).

4.3 Gastritis

4.3.1 Acute vs. Chronic

Gastritis refers to **inflammation** of the stomach lining:

1. **Acute Gastritis**
   - Often erosive, triggered by **stress** (critical illness), **alcohol**, **NSAIDs**, or infection.
   - Sudden onset with possible epigastric pain, nausea, or vomiting.
2. **Chronic Gastritis**
   - Prolonged inflammation; can be **non-erosive** (like autoimmune gastritis or H. pylori) or erosive.
   - May progress to atrophic gastritis (loss of gastric glands, risk of B12 deficiency) or intestinal metaplasia.

4.3.2 Erosive vs. Non-Erosive

1. **Erosive Gastritis**
   - Causes superficial ulcers or erosions.
   - Common triggers: alcohol binge, systemic stress (ICU patients).
2. **Non-Erosive**
   - Autoimmune (parietal cell antibodies → pernicious anemia), H. pylori infiltration.
   - Less mucosal destruction on endoscopy but can have deep changes microscopically.

4.3.3 Management

- **Remove/Reduce Offending Factors**: Alcohol, NSAIDs, smoking.
- **Medications**: PPIs or H2 blockers for acid reduction, sucralfate for mucosal protection.
- **H. pylori Eradication**: If present, treat as in PUD.
- **Autoimmune**: Monitor B12 levels, potential pernicious anemia.

4.4 Barrett's Esophagus

4.4.1 Metaplastic Change

Barrett's esophagus occurs when **chronic GERD** stimulates metaplasia in the distal esophagus lining, replacing normal stratified squamous epithelium with columnar epithelium resembling the intestine:

1. **Why It Develops**
   - Prolonged acid reflux injures the lower esophageal tissue.
   - The body attempts to adapt by adopting a more acid-resistant type of epithelium.
2. **Cancer Risk**
   - Increases the risk of **esophageal adenocarcinoma**; though absolute risk is

relatively low, it's significantly higher than in non-Barrett's patients.

- Dysplasia grading (low-grade, high-grade) signals progressive malignant changes.

4.4.2 Surveillance Endoscopies

1. **Diagnostic**:
   - Endoscopy sees a salmon-colored lining extending above the gastroesophageal junction. Biopsy confirms intestinal-type columnar cells.
2. **Follow-Up**:
   - Periodic endoscopies check for dysplasia. Frequency depends on the presence/grade of dysplasia (e.g., 3–5 years if no dysplasia, more frequent if low-grade).
   - **Endoscopic Mucosal Resection or Ablation (RFA)** for high-grade dysplasia to prevent carcinoma progression.
3. **Lifestyle & Treatment**
   - Aggressive management of reflux (PPI therapy, potential surgical fundoplication).
   - Lifestyle modifications (weight loss, avoiding trigger foods) to reduce acid exposure.

4.5 Key Terms Recap

- **GERD (Gastroesophageal Reflux Disease)**: Acid reflux due to LES weakness, leading to heartburn, regurgitation, possible esophagitis.
- **Peptic Ulcer Disease (PUD)**: Ulcers in the stomach/duodenum commonly linked to H. pylori or NSAIDs.
- **H. pylori**: A bacterium colonizing the stomach, implicated in ulcers and some gastric cancers.
- **Gastritis**: Inflammation of the gastric lining, which can be acute or chronic, erosive or non-erosive.
- **Barrett's Esophagus**: Metaplastic change in the lower esophagus from chronic acid exposure, raising risk for adenocarcinoma.
- **PPI (Proton Pump Inhibitor)**: Potently decreases gastric acid secretion (e.g., omeprazole, lansoprazole).

4.6 Quick Quiz

1. **Multiple Choice**: Which factor is **most strongly** associated with duodenal ulcer formation?
   a) Alcohol abuse
   b) Helicobacter pylori
   c) Corticosteroid overuse
   d) Excess fiber intake

2. **True or False**: Gastritis can be caused by both erosive factors (like NSAIDs) and non-erosive factors (like autoimmunity or H. pylori).

3. **Fill in the Blank**: **Barrett's esophagus** involves a metaplastic change from normal _____ epithelium to a columnar type, predominantly due to chronic acid reflux.

4. **Which medication category is considered the mainstay treatment for healing erosive esophagitis and ulcers by markedly reducing stomach acid?**

   a) Antacids

   b) H2 receptor blockers

   c) Proton pump inhibitors

   d) Sucralfate

5. **Short Answer**: List two key lifestyle modifications helpful in managing GERD.

Answers

1. **(b) Helicobacter pylori** – A common cause of duodenal ulcers.

2. **True** – Erosive (drugs, alcohol) or non-erosive (autoimmune, H. pylori) can provoke gastritis.

3. **Stratified squamous** – Barrett's replaces it with a columnar (intestinal-like) lining.

4. **(c) Proton pump inhibitors** – They profoundly decrease acid secretion, promoting mucosal healing.
5. **Example**: "Weight loss if overweight, avoiding late-night meals, propping up head of bed, reducing trigger foods (acidic/spicy/fatty)."

Concluding Perspective

From the **burning** retrosternal discomfort of **GERD** to the gnawing epigastric pain of **peptic ulcers**, upper GI disorders often revolve around **excess acid, damaged mucosal defenses**, or **bacterial colonization (H. pylori)**. **Gastritis** is a broader label for stomach lining inflammation, and **Barrett's esophagus** underscores the potential for chronic reflux to escalate into precancerous conditions.

With these fundamentals in place, **Chapter 5** takes us onward into the **Small Intestine & Malabsorption Syndromes**, exploring celiac disease, the intricacies of nutrient absorption, and how seemingly minor changes in the small bowel can lead to major deficiencies or health challenges.

Chapter 5: Small Intestine & Malabsorption Syndromes

5.1 The Small Intestine's Role in Nutrient Absorption

5.1.1 Overview of Structure & Function

The **small intestine** is the primary site of **digestion and absorption** within the GI tract. Its three segments—**duodenum, jejunum**, and **ileum**—work in sequence to:

1. **Break Down Nutrients**
   ○ Pancreatic enzymes, bile salts, and brush border enzymes transform carbohydrates, proteins, and fats into absorbable units (monosaccharides, amino acids, fatty acids, glycerol).

2. **Maximize Surface Area**
   ○ **Villi** (finger-like projections) and **microvilli** (tiny projections on enterocytes) create a "brush border," dramatically expanding the mucosal surface for nutrient uptake.

3. **Transport to the Body**

○ Absorbed nutrients enter the bloodstream (carbohydrates, proteins) or the lymphatic system (lipids via chylomicrons) to fuel tissues throughout the body.

5.1.2 Key Points in Physiology

- **Duodenum**: Receives **bile** and **pancreatic juices** that neutralize acidic chyme and facilitate fat digestion.
- **Jejunum**: Major site for absorbing most nutrients (carbs, proteins, minerals).
- **Ileum**: Critical for **vitamin B_{12}** and **bile salt** reabsorption.
- **Enterocytes**: The absorptive cells lining the villi, turnover is frequent; damage to these cells can quickly impair nutrient uptake.

Malabsorption occurs when structural damage (villous atrophy, resection) or functional deficits (lack of enzymes, poor motility) hamper nutrient absorption, leading to symptoms like diarrhea, weight loss, and nutritional deficiencies.

5.2 Celiac Disease

5.2.1 Immune-Mediated Reaction to Gluten

Celiac disease (also called **gluten-sensitive enteropathy** or **celiac sprue**) arises from an **immune response** in genetically predisposed individuals to **gluten** proteins found in wheat, barley, and rye. This reaction triggers **villous atrophy** in the small intestine, resulting in malabsorption and systemic effects.

1. **Pathophysiology**
   - **Gluten** is partially digested into peptides (gliadin fractions). In celiac, these peptides elicit a T-cell–mediated inflammatory response in the **duodenum**/jejunum.
   - Chronic inflammation destroys **villi**, flattening the mucosa, reducing absorptive surface.
2. **Genetic & Environmental Factors**
   - Strong association with **HLA-DQ2** or **HLA-DQ8** haplotypes.
   - Environmental triggers (gastrointestinal infections, changes in gut microbiota) can unmask or worsen celiac in susceptible individuals.

5.2.2 Symptoms & Presentation

1. **Classic Malabsorption**
   - **Diarrhea**, **steatorrhea** (fatty stools), abdominal bloating, weight loss.
   - Children may show failure to thrive or delayed growth.
2. **Extraintestinal Manifestations**

- Dermatitis herpetiformis: Intensely pruritic skin rash with blisters.
- Iron-deficiency anemia (chronic blood or nutrient loss), osteopenia (vitamin D and calcium malabsorption).
- Neurologic symptoms (peripheral neuropathy) in some severe cases.

3. **Silent & Atypical Celiac**
- Some have minimal GI symptoms but exhibit iron deficiency, fatigue, or mild anemia.
- Detected by screening in relatives of confirmed celiac patients.

5.2.3 Diagnostic Testing

1. **Serological Tests**
- **tTG-IgA (Tissue Transglutaminase Antibody):** First-line screening test, high sensitivity.
- **EMA (Endomysial Antibody):** Highly specific, used to confirm uncertain tTG results.
- Ensure normal total IgA levels to avoid false negatives if IgA deficient.

2. **Endoscopic Biopsy**
- **Gold standard** for confirming celiac. Duodenal biopsy typically shows villous atrophy, crypt

hyperplasia, and increased intraepithelial lymphocytes.

- o Biopsies can also distinguish refractory sprue, tropical sprue, or other causes of villous damage.

3. **Genetic Testing**
   - o **HLA-DQ2/DQ8** positivity is common but not diagnostic alone—negativity essentially rules out celiac.

5.2.4 Gluten-Free Diet & Management

1. **Dietary Intervention**
   - o A **strict gluten-free diet (GFD)** is central. Even trace gluten can maintain inflammation.
   - o Rechallenge or accidental exposure can trigger relapse.

2. **Nutritional Supplementation**
   - o Iron, calcium, vitamin D, B_{12} if deficiencies exist.

3. **Monitoring**
   - o Serology (tTG-IgA) can track dietary adherence and mucosal healing.
   - o Incomplete improvement may suggest **refractory celiac** or hidden gluten exposure.

5.3 Tropical Sprue & Other Malabsorption

5.3.1 Tropical Sprue

Tropical sprue mimics celiac but occurs in tropical regions (Caribbean, South Asia). Key distinctions:

1. **Etiology**
   - Possibly an **infectious or environmental** trigger, leading to chronic inflammation in the small bowel.
   - Different from **tropical enteropathy** (subclinical) by severity and malabsorption.
2. **Symptoms**
   - Chronic diarrhea, malabsorption of folate/B_{12}, leading to megaloblastic anemia.
   - Weight loss, bloating, fatigue.
3. **Diagnosis & Treatment**
   - Exclusion of other causes like celiac (serologies negative), travel or residence history in endemic areas.
   - Broad-spectrum antibiotics (tetracycline), plus supplementation (folate, B_{12}).

5.3.2 Other Malabsorption Syndromes

1. **Whipple's Disease**

- **Tropheryma whipplei** infection, rare but can cause systemic issues (arthralgias, cardiac/neurologic).
- Intestinal biopsy shows periodic acid–Schiff (PAS)-positive macrophages.

2. **Giardiasis**
   - Protozoan parasite (Giardia lamblia) colonizes duodenum.
   - Foul-smelling, greasy stools, often contracted from contaminated water.
   - Metronidazole or tinidazole typically cures it.

5.4 Short Bowel Syndrome

5.4.1 Causes & Consequences

Short bowel syndrome (SBS) arises from **extensive surgical resection** of the small intestine (e.g., due to Crohn's complications or infarction) or congenital anomalies. With **less absorptive surface**, patients struggle with:

1. **Malabsorption** of macronutrients, vitamins, minerals.
2. **Diarrhea** and **dehydration** if fluids aren't managed adequately.
3. **Weight Loss & Malnutrition**, possible metabolic derangements.

5.4.2 Management Approaches

1. **Nutritional Support**
   - **Parenteral Nutrition (TPN)** if severely reduced bowel length.
   - High-calorie, nutrient-dense diets, sometimes specialized enteral formulas.
2. **Medications**
   - **Antimotility** agents (loperamide) slow transit, improving nutrient contact time.
   - **Teduglutide** (GLP-2 analog) can aid adaptation by promoting mucosal growth.
3. **Adaptation & Surgery**
   - The remaining bowel often undergoes "adaptation," lengthening villi to improve absorption.
   - Intestinal transplant is a last resort if TPN complications or absolute shortage of bowel persist.

5.5 Clinical Approach: Diagnostic Tools & Interventions

5.5.1 D-xylose Test & Stool Fat Quantification

1. **D-xylose Test**

- Evaluates **mucosal** absorption ability in the proximal small intestine. Low urinary excretion suggests mucosal damage (celiac, tropical sprue).

2. **Stool Fat Quantification**
   - A 72-hour stool collection measuring fat excretion indicates **steatorrhea**. High levels confirm fat malabsorption (pancreatic insufficiency, small bowel disease).

5.5.2 Dietary & Pharmacologic Interventions

1. **Dietary Measures**
   - **Gluten-Free Diet** for celiac, **lactose restriction** for lactose intolerance.
   - High-calorie, high-protein for short bowel syndrome; specialized elemental feeds if needed.
2. **Vitamin & Mineral Supplementation**
   - B_{12} in ileal resection or celiac, fat-soluble vitamins (A, D, E, K) if steatorrhea.
3. **Pancreatic Enzyme Replacement**
   - If exocrine pancreatic insufficiency is an issue (chronic pancreatitis or resection).

5.6 Key Terms Recap

- **Villous Atrophy**: Loss of normal intestinal villi height, reducing absorption (e.g., celiac).
- **Steatorrhea**: Excess fat in stools, indicating fat malabsorption.
- **Dermatitis Herpetiformis**: Itchy blistering rash associated with celiac disease.
- **Tropical Sprue**: Malabsorption in tropical regions, responding to antibiotics and supplements.
- **Short Bowel Syndrome**: Bowel length insufficient for normal nutrient/water absorption, often needing TPN.

5.7 Quick Quiz

1. **Multiple Choice**: Which organism is strongly linked to peptic ulcers yet *not* typically associated with small-intestine malabsorption syndromes?
   a) Giardia lamblia
   b) Helicobacter pylori
   c) Tropheryma whipplei
   d) Trichinella spiralis
2. **True or False**: A gluten-free diet is the **primary** treatment approach for celiac disease.
3. **Fill in the Blank**: _____ is a T-cell–mediated disease causing villous atrophy in response to dietary gluten, frequently presenting with diarrhea, malabsorption, and sometimes dermatitis herpetiformis.

4. **Which of the following is most associated with "megalo-blastic" anemia due to folate or B_{12} malabsorption in tropical regions?**

   a) Giardiasis

   b) Tropical sprue

   c) Lactose intolerance

   d) Irritable bowel syndrome

5. **Short Answer**: Provide one key management strategy for **short bowel syndrome** and explain its importance.

Answers

1. **(b) Helicobacter pylori** – Typically causes gastric/duodenal ulcers, not small-bowel malabsorption issues.

2. **True** – Eliminating gluten halts the immune-driven damage in celiac disease.

3. **Celiac disease** – Marked by mucosal changes triggered by gluten.

4. **(b) Tropical sprue** – Infectious or environmental cause in tropical areas, often leading to B_{12}/folate deficiency.

5. **Example**: "Use of parenteral nutrition (TPN) in severe short bowel syndrome ensures adequate caloric and nutrient intake when the remaining bowel can't meet requirements."

Final Thoughts

The **small intestine** serves as the body's main nutrient gateway, so disorders like **celiac disease** or **tropical sprue** can undercut energy supply and lead to systemic deficits. **Short bowel syndrome** underscores how the length—and health—of intestinal mucosa is pivotal. By employing specialized tests (D-xylose, stool fat analysis) and interventions (dietary modifications, nutritional support, or medications), most malabsorption syndromes can be managed or significantly improved. In **Chapter 6**, we move on to **Inflammatory Bowel Disease (IBD): Crohn's & Ulcerative Colitis**, exploring autoimmune-driven inflammation that can strike anywhere from the mouth to the anus, with wide-ranging impacts on absorption and bowel function.

Chapter 6: Inflammatory Bowel Disease (IBD) — Crohn's & Ulcerative Colitis

6.1 IBD Overview

6.1.1 What Defines IBD?

Inflammatory Bowel Disease (IBD) is a term encompassing **chronic, relapsing-remitting inflammatory disorders** of the gastrointestinal tract. The two primary subtypes:

- **Crohn's Disease**
- **Ulcerative Colitis (UC)**

They differ in **location**, **depth of inflammation**, and **clinical** and **endoscopic** findings. Both can lead to significant morbidity without proper diagnosis and therapy.

6.1.2 Underlying Mechanisms

Though the exact causes remain partially unknown, IBD likely arises from:

1. **Genetic Susceptibility**
   - Certain HLA haplotypes, NOD2 mutations (in Crohn's).
   - Family history increases risk for either form of IBD.
2. **Immune Dysregulation**
   - Overactive immune responses to gut flora or dietary antigens.
   - T-cell–mediated process, with different cytokine profiles in Crohn's vs. UC.
3. **Environmental Factors**
   - Westernized diets, smoking (aggravates Crohn's but may somewhat protect against UC), and possibly gut microbiome alterations.

6.2 Crohn's Disease

6.2.1 Transmural Inflammation & "Skip Lesions"

Crohn's disease can affect **any part** of the GI tract, from the mouth to the anus, though the **terminal ileum** and **perianal region** are common sites. Key features:

1. **Transmural Inflammation**
   - Spans the entire thickness of the bowel wall (mucosa through serosa).

- o Leads to complications like **fistulas** and **strictures**.

2. **Skip Lesions**
   - o Discontinuous involvement: inflamed segments interspersed with normal regions.
   - o Endoscopy may reveal "cobblestone" appearance, with deep ulcers and fissures.

6.2.2 Clinical Manifestations

1. **Symptoms**
   - o **Diarrhea** (often non-bloody unless colonic involvement), abdominal pain (often right lower quadrant if ileum is affected), weight loss, fever during flares.
   - o Perianal disease: fistulas, abscesses, anal fissures cause local discomfort, drainage.

2. **Complications**
   - o **Strictures** can obstruct the bowel, leading to cramping, bloating, vomiting.
   - o **Fistulas** may form abnormal channels between bowel loops or to other organs (bladder, vagina) or the skin.

6.2.3 Special Considerations

- • **Smoking** typically worsens Crohn's activity.

- **Malabsorption** can occur if the small bowel is heavily diseased or resected (B_{12} deficiency if ileum is impacted).
- **Growth Failure** or delayed puberty in children if onset is early.

6.3 Ulcerative Colitis (UC)

6.3.1 Mucosal Inflammation & Continuous Pattern

Ulcerative Colitis is limited to the **colon and rectum**, involving only the **mucosal layer**:

1. **Rectal Involvement**
   - UC always starts in the **rectum** and extends proximally in a **continuous** (non-skip) fashion.
   - Can be proctitis (rectum only), left-sided colitis, or pancolitis (entire colon).
2. **Superficial Lesions**
   - Inflammatory changes typically confined to mucosa (and submucosa in severe cases).
   - Deeper layers remain unaffected, so fistulas and strictures are less common than in Crohn's.

6.3.2 Clinical Presentation

1. **Bloody Diarrhea**

- Hallmark symptom, often with mucus.
- Frequent small-volume bowel movements, urgency, and tenesmus if rectum is heavily inflamed.

2. **Severity Spectrum**
   - **Mild**: <4 stools/day, minimal systemic impact.
   - **Severe**: >6 bloody stools/day, systemic signs (fever, tachycardia), risk of toxic megacolon.

3. **Risk of Colon Cancer**
   - Chronic mucosal inflammation over many years (especially pancolitis) significantly raises **colorectal cancer** risk.
   - Surveillance colonoscopies recommended after 8–10 years of disease.

6.3.3 Extraintestinal Manifestations

Both Crohn's and UC can have **systemic manifestations**:

- **Arthritis** (peripheral or axial), sacroiliitis.
- **Skin lesions** (erythema nodosum, pyoderma gangrenosum).
- **Eye** involvement (uveitis, scleritis).
- **Liver** (primary sclerosing cholangitis more common with UC).

6.4 Diagnosis & Therapy

6.4.1 Diagnostic Workup

1. **Colonoscopy & Biopsy**
   - Reveals distribution of lesions (continuous vs. skip), extent, and histology.
   - UC: Inflammation mostly limited to mucosa, "pseudopolyps," continuous starting from rectum.
   - Crohn's: Patchy involvement, deep linear ulcers, transmural inflammation.
2. **Stool Markers & Labs**
   - **Fecal calprotectin** or lactoferrin: Elevated in active inflammation (differentiating IBD from IBS).
   - **ESR, CRP** for systemic inflammation.
   - **Nutritional deficiencies** (iron, B_{12}, folate) if absorption is compromised.
3. **Imaging**
   - **MR enterography** or small bowel follow-through for Crohn's (assessing strictures, fistulas).
   - **CT scan** in acute severe flares to check for complications (abscess, perforation).

6.4.2 Medical Management

1. **Corticosteroids**
   - Treat flares (acute attacks) effectively.

- Not ideal for long-term maintenance due to side effects (osteoporosis, hyperglycemia, adrenal suppression).

2. **Immunomodulators**
   - **Azathioprine, 6-mercaptopurine, methotrexate**: Maintain remission in moderate-to-severe cases.
   - Slow onset of action but can spare steroid usage.

3. **Biologics**
   - **Anti-TNF Agents** (infliximab, adalimumab) for moderate-severe Crohn's/UC.
   - Other classes: Anti-integrins (vedolizumab) or IL-12/23 inhibitors (ustekinumab).
   - Tailored to disease severity, location, patient's comorbidities.

4. **Aminosalicylates (5-ASA)**
   - Mesalamine or sulfasalazine for mild-moderate UC, less effective in Crohn's except for colonic disease involvement.

6.4.3 Surgical Options

1. **Crohn's Surgery**
   - Address complications (strictures, fistulas, abscesses).

- Resection of severely diseased bowel but mindful of short bowel syndrome risk with repeated resections.
- Surgery is **not** curative; disease can recur in remaining GI segments.

2. **UC Surgery**
   - **Proctocolectomy** (removal of colon and rectum) is **curative** for UC (removing the entire diseased organ).
   - Ileal pouch-anal anastomosis (IPAA) can maintain defecatory control.
   - Indicated for refractory disease, severe complications, or dysplasia/cancer risk.

6.5 Key Terms Recap

- **Transmural**: Inflammation spanning the entire bowel wall thickness (Crohn's).
- **Skip Lesions**: Patchy areas of disease with normal segments in between (Crohn's).
- **Continuous Colonic Involvement**: Mucosal disease extending from rectum proximally without gaps (UC).
- **Strictures & Fistulas**: Common Crohn's complications due to deeper tissue injury.
- **Pancolitis**: UC involving the entire colon; heightens colon cancer risk.

- **Immunomodulators**: Drugs like azathioprine reducing immune-driven inflammation; can maintain remission.
- **Anti-TNF Agents**: Biologic therapy (infliximab, adalimumab) effective in moderate-severe IBD.

6.6 Quick Quiz

1. **Multiple Choice**: Which statement **best** differentiates Crohn's disease from ulcerative colitis?
   a) Both are limited to the colon.
   b) Crohn's is confined to mucosal inflammation while UC has transmural involvement.
   c) Crohn's can cause skip lesions and affects any GI segment; UC is continuous and limited to the colon.
   d) Smoking helps Crohn's but worsens UC.
2. **True or False**: Surgery can be **curative** for Crohn's disease.
3. **Fill in the Blank**: Ulcerative colitis primarily affects the _____ layer, beginning in the rectum and extending proximally in a continuous manner.
4. **Which medication class is often used first-line to quickly quell moderate-severe IBD flares but is not recommended for prolonged maintenance due to side effects?**
   a) Aminosalicylates (5-ASA)
   b) Corticosteroids

c) Anti-TNF agents

d) Antibiotics

5. **Short Answer**: In mild ulcerative colitis, what is one common medication used to maintain remission, and why might it be less effective in Crohn's disease?

Answers

1. **(c) Crohn's can cause skip lesions and affect any GI segment; UC is continuous and limited to the colon** – Summarizes the essential difference.
2. **False** – Surgery is not curative for Crohn's; disease may recur in remaining bowel. UC, on the other hand, can be cured by proctocolectomy.
3. **Mucosal** – UC typically involves the mucosa (and sometimes submucosa).
4. **(b) Corticosteroids** – Highly effective for acute flares but not suitable long-term due to systemic side effects.
5. **Example**: "Mesalamine (5-ASA). It's useful in mild UC for mucosal inflammation control but less effective for Crohn's because Crohn's often involves deeper layers and skip areas not well-targeted by 5-ASA therapy."

Concluding Note

Inflammatory Bowel Disease embodies an intersection of **immune dysregulation**, **genetic predisposition**, and

environmental influences, culminating in chronic GI inflammation. **Crohn's disease** can arise anywhere with patchy, transmural lesions, while **ulcerative colitis** remains limited to the colon's mucosal layer. Though no single cure exists for Crohn's, modern **immunosuppressants** and **biologic therapies** greatly improve outcomes. In UC, **surgery** can be curative but is typically reserved for refractory cases or when there's a high cancer risk. With an appreciation of IBD's complexities, we pivot next to **Chapter 7**, addressing **Irritable Bowel Syndrome (IBS)** and other functional GI disorders, which, while not inflammatory, still cause substantial patient distress and require distinct management approaches.

Chapter 7: Irritable Bowel Syndrome (IBS) & Functional Disorders

7.1 Understanding Functional GI Syndromes

7.1.1 Defining "Functional" Disorders

Functional GI disorders are those in which **chronic symptoms**—such as abdominal pain, altered bowel habits, or bloating—occur **without** obvious structural or biochemical abnormalities detectable by routine tests. This contrasts with organic diseases (e.g., IBD, ulcers) that exhibit clear endoscopic or histologic changes.

1. **Brain–Gut Axis**
   - The GI tract and central nervous system maintain bidirectional communication.
   - Stress, anxiety, or depression can intensify GI symptoms; conversely, GI distress can worsen stress or mood.
2. **Biopsychosocial Model**

○ Recognizes psychological, social, and physiological factors in causing or perpetuating disorders like IBS.

7.1.2 The Role of IBS in Functional Disorders

Among functional GI issues, **Irritable Bowel Syndrome (IBS)** stands out as **common** and **chronic**, affecting daily life for millions of patients worldwide. It's a prime example of how symptoms can be **debilitating**, yet endoscopy or imaging appear relatively normal.

7.2 IBS Subtypes

7.2.1 Diarrhea-Predominant (IBS-D)

Patients with **IBS-D** experience:

- **Frequent Loose Stools**: Often urgent, sometimes triggered by meals or stress.
- **Abdominal Pain** relieved by defecation or passing gas.
- **Potential Bloating** and discomfort vary day to day.

7.2.2 Constipation-Predominant (IBS-C)

IBS-C involves:

- **Infrequent, Hard, or Lumpy Stools**.

- **Straining** during bowel movements, incomplete evacuation feeling.
- **Abdominal Pain/Bloating** may fluctuate with bowel habit changes.

7.2.3 Mixed (IBS-M)

Many people oscillate between **diarrhea and constipation**, sometimes unpredictably:

- Episodes of **loose stools** and **constipation** in alternating cycles.
- Symptom shifts can be confusing, complicating management and dietary approaches.

*(Note: Some categorize **IBS-U** (unclassified) for individuals not neatly fitting these subtypes.)*

7.3 Pathophysiology & Triggers

7.3.1 Brain–Gut Axis & Stress

IBS is often explained via a disrupted **brain–gut axis**, where signals between the enteric nervous system and central nervous system are **oversensitive**:

- **Visceral Hypersensitivity**: Patients may perceive normal intestinal contractions or gas as painful.

- **Stress & Emotional Factors**: Anxiety or depression can heighten symptoms, while chronic GI discomfort can increase stress—creating a cycle.

7.3.2 Diet & FODMAPs

FODMAPs—fermentable oligosaccharides, disaccharides, monosaccharides, and polyols—are carbohydrates that:

- **Ferment** in the colon, producing gas and osmotic fluid shifts.
- Common culprits: high-fructose fruits, lactose (milk), certain vegetables (onion, garlic), and sugar alcohols (sorbitol, mannitol).
- A **low-FODMAP diet** can reduce bloating, cramping, and stool irregularities in many IBS sufferers.

7.3.3 Abdominal Pain Relieved by Defecation

One hallmark IBS feature is **pain alleviation** after bowel movements:

- Reflects the **functional** nature of IBS, where motility or hypersensitivity underlies discomfort rather than structural lesions.
- Patients often describe a "cramping" that eases upon passing stool or gas.

7.4 Diagnosis (Rome IV Criteria)

7.4.1 Symptom-Based Classification

The **Rome IV Criteria** for IBS diagnosis emphasize **recurrent abdominal pain**, on average at least 1 day per week in the last 3 months, associated with **two or more** of:

1. **Relation to Defecation** (pain improvement or worsening after a bowel movement).
2. **Change in Frequency** of stool.
3. **Change in Form (Appearance)** of stool.

Symptoms should start at least 6 months before diagnosis. This clinical method helps differentiate IBS from organic diseases, although "red flag" signs (alarm features) still warrant further investigations.

7.4.2 Excluding Organic Pathology

1. **Alarm Features**
   - Significant weight loss, GI bleeding, persistent fever, anemia, nocturnal symptoms.
   - These raise suspicion for IBD, malignancies, or celiac.
2. **Lab & Imaging**

- Normal inflammatory markers (CRP, ESR), negative fecal calprotectin often point away from IBD.
- Negative colonoscopy or imaging further supports a functional disorder if alarm signs are absent.

Note: Testing for celiac disease or other malabsorption syndromes may be prudent, given overlapping symptoms (bloating, diarrhea).

7.5 Management Strategies

7.5.1 Dietary Modifications

1. **Low-FODMAP Diet**
   - Temporarily limiting fermentable carbs (e.g., wheat, onions, certain fruits) can alleviate bloating, gas, abdominal pain.
   - Reintroduce systematically to identify specific triggers.
2. **Fiber**
   - **Soluble fiber** (psyllium) may help IBS-C by normalizing stool consistency.
   - **Insoluble fiber** (bran) can exacerbate symptoms for some. Gradual introduction is recommended.

3. **Hydration & Regular Meals**
    - Adequate fluids help bowel motility.
    - Smaller, frequent meals reduce over-distension and cramping.

7.5.2 Pharmacological Aids

1. **Antispasmodics (Anticholinergics)**
    - Dicyclomine, hyoscyamine reduce intestinal smooth muscle spasm, easing cramping.
    - Potential side effects: dry mouth, constipation, blurred vision.
2. **Laxatives or Stool Softeners**
    - Useful in IBS-C to relieve constipation.
    - *e.g., polyethylene glycol (PEG), lactulose (though can cause bloating).*
3. **Antidiarrheals**
    - Loperamide for IBS-D, decreasing stool frequency and urgency.
    - Doesn't always address pain or bloating.
4. **Low-Dose Antidepressants**
    - **Tricyclics (TCAs)** or **SSRIs** can modulate pain perception via the brain–gut axis.
    - TCAs (e.g., amitriptyline) beneficial for IBS-D; SSRIs sometimes help IBS-C or coexisting depression/anxiety.

7.5.3 Psychological Therapies

1. **Cognitive Behavioral Therapy (CBT)**
   - Addresses anxiety, maladaptive thoughts, and coping strategies.
   - Patients often learn relaxation techniques, problem-solving skills to lessen symptom severity.
2. **Gut-Directed Hypnotherapy**
   - Shows promise in reducing visceral hypersensitivity, stress-driven flare-ups.
3. **Stress Reduction & Support**
   - Yoga, mindfulness-based programs, or counseling can improve overall quality of life.

7.6 Key Terms Recap

- **Functional Disorder**: Chronic symptoms without overt structural or biochemical abnormalities (e.g., IBS).
- **IBS-D, IBS-C, IBS-M**: IBS variants (diarrhea, constipation, or mixed).
- **Rome IV Criteria**: Diagnostic tool for IBS based on stool changes, pain frequency, relation to defecation.
- **FODMAPs**: Fermentable carbohydrates that can trigger bloating and discomfort in IBS.

- **Visceral Hypersensitivity**: Heightened perception of normal gut sensations, central to IBS pathophysiology.
- **CBT (Cognitive Behavioral Therapy)**: Psychological approach aiding in symptom control for functional GI disorders.

7.7 Quick Quiz

1. **Multiple Choice**: Which hallmark is **most strongly** associated with IBS?
   a) Continuous bloody diarrhea
   b) Nocturnal severe pain awakening patients
   c) Abdominal pain relieved by defecation
   d) Perianal fistula formation
2. **True or False**: IBS often presents with **alarm features** like significant weight loss, anemia, or overt GI bleeding.
3. **Fill in the Blank**: **FODMAPs** are fermentable carbohydrates that can exacerbate IBS symptoms by increasing _____ and fluid shifts in the colon.
4. **Which diet approach is frequently used to help patients with IBS identify specific trigger foods and reduce gas/bloating?**
   a) Ketogenic diet
   b) Low-FODMAP diet

c) High-protein diet

d) Gluten-free diet

5. **Short Answer**: Name one common pharmacologic therapy for IBS-D and briefly explain its main effect.

Answers

1. **(c) Abdominal pain relieved by defecation** – A key IBS symptom as per Rome IV.
2. **False** – Alarm features suggest an **organic** disease; IBS typically lacks them.
3. **Gas** – FODMAPs ferment, increasing gas production and water content in the intestines.
4. **(b) Low-FODMAP diet** – Widely adopted for IBS symptom control.
5. **Example**: "Loperamide, an antidiarrheal that slows gut motility and helps reduce stool frequency and urgency in IBS-D."

Final Note

While **IBS** can cause significant life disruption—pain, erratic bowel habits, bloating—unlike inflammatory or structural GI diseases, it doesn't typically lead to **permanent damage**. Tackling dietary triggers (like **FODMAPs**), addressing stress, and using targeted medications (antispasmodics, laxatives, or antidiarrheals) can transform symptom burden dramatically. In

Chapter 8, we'll shift to **Colorectal Diseases & Screening**, analyzing how polyps, diverticular disease, and colon cancer risk shape clinical recommendations for colonoscopies and preventive measures. By contrasting IBS with organic colonic disorders, the importance of identifying **red flags** that suggest deeper pathology becomes clearer.

Chapter 8: Colorectal Diseases & Screening

8.1 Colorectal Polyps

8.1.1 Adenomatous vs. Hyperplastic Polyps

Colorectal polyps are growths projecting from the colonic mucosal surface, varying in shape (sessile, pedunculated) and malignant potential:

1. **Adenomatous Polyps (Adenomas)**
   - Precancerous lesions that can progress to **adenocarcinoma** via the **adenoma–carcinoma sequence** if not removed.
   - Histological subtypes: tubular, tubulovillous, villous (villous often has higher malignant risk).
   - Larger polyps (>1 cm) and those with dysplasia are more likely to harbor or develop malignancy.
2. **Hyperplastic Polyps**
   - Typically **non-neoplastic**, often found in the distal colon and rectum.
   - Usually small (<5 mm) and carry minimal or no malignant potential unless they are large or part

of a "sessile serrated" pattern (which can have some risk).

3. **Sessile Serrated Polyps**
   - Morphologically appear "hyperplastic" but can have molecular changes (serrated pathway) leading to cancer if left untreated.
   - Emphasizes the need for careful pathologic evaluation.

8.1.2 Polypectomy for Prevention

1. **Colonoscopy**:
   - The gold standard for identifying and removing polyps.
   - Polyps discovered during screening are typically resected via a snare or forceps biopsy (polypectomy), reducing future cancer risk.
2. **Surveillance**:
   - Follow-up colonoscopy intervals depend on polyp number, size, and histopathology (e.g., adenoma with high-grade dysplasia might require earlier re-check).
3. **Genetic Syndromes**
   - Familial Adenomatous Polyposis (FAP), Lynch syndrome (HNPCC) cause numerous or early

polyps; more frequent endoscopic surveillance recommended.

8.2 Colon Cancer

8.2.1 Symptoms & Alarm Features

Colorectal cancer arises when mutations accumulate in polyp cells or from a separate malignant focus. Common presentations:

1. **Rectal Bleeding**
   - Visible red blood on the stool or hidden (occult) blood.
   - Could indicate lower GI lesions if bright red, but any unexplained bleeding is concerning.
2. **Altered Bowel Habits**
   - Persistent diarrhea or constipation, narrower stools (if a mass partially obstructs the lumen).
   - Patients might describe a sensation of incomplete evacuation.
3. **Alarm Features**
   - **Unexplained Weight Loss**: Could signal advanced disease or systemic impact.
   - **Anemia** (particularly iron deficiency in older adults) raising suspicion of chronic blood loss.

○ **Weakness, Fatigue** from ongoing bleeding.

8.2.2 Staging & Treatment Approaches

1. **Imaging & Colonoscopy**
   ○ **Colonoscopy** confirms lesions, allows biopsy.
   ○ **CT scan, MRI** for local or distant staging (liver, lung metastases).
2. **TNM Classification**
   ○ **T** indicates tumor infiltration depth (into bowel wall layers).
   ○ **N** shows lymph node involvement.
   ○ **M** reveals distant metastasis.
3. **Surgery**
   ○ **Localized Disease (Stage I or II)**: Resection of the tumor-bearing segment (colectomy) with adjacent lymph nodes. Potentially curative if no spread.
   ○ **More Advanced (Stage III or IV)**: Still consider resection, possibly combined with chemo (fluorouracil, oxaliplatin) or targeted therapies.
4. **Chemotherapy & Targeted Therapies**
   ○ **Adjuvant Chemo** post-surgery in stage III or high-risk stage II.

- Biologic Agents (e.g., bevacizumab targeting VEGF, cetuximab targeting EGFR) for metastatic disease.
- Immunotherapy: Checkpoint inhibitors in select cases with microsatellite instability (MSI-high).

8.3 Diverticular Disease

8.3.1 Diverticulosis vs. Diverticulitis

Diverticula are small pouch-like protrusions of the colonic wall (commonly in the sigmoid colon). Risk factors include age, low-fiber diets, and chronic constipation.

1. Diverticulosis
   - Presence of diverticula, often asymptomatic or mild bloating/irregular bowel habits.
   - Can result in painless bleeding (diverticular hemorrhage) if a diverticulum erodes a blood vessel.
2. Diverticulitis
   - Infection/inflammation of a diverticulum, potentially causing left lower quadrant pain, fever, and altered bowel habits.

- Ranges from mild (treated with oral antibiotics, diet adjustment) to severe (complicated by abscess, perforation, peritonitis).

8.3.2 Risk Factors & Complications

1. **Low-Fiber Diet**
   - May lead to higher intraluminal pressures and outpouching.
2. **Age**
   - Prevalence increases over 50 years, with more or larger diverticula forming.
3. **Complications**
   - **Diverticular Bleeding**: Usually painless, can be brisk.
   - **Abscess**: Localized infected fluid; may need drainage.
   - **Fistula**: Rarely, inflamed diverticulum forms a tract to other organs (bladder, vagina) or skin.

8.3.3 Management

- **Uncomplicated Diverticulitis**: Outpatient antibiotics (covering anaerobes, gram-negatives) plus a low-residue or liquid diet short-term, then high-fiber diet for prevention.

- **Complicated Cases**: IV antibiotics, possible surgical resection if perforation or recurrent severe episodes.
- **Prevention**: High-fiber intake, adequate fluids, regular exercise.

8.4 Screening Guidelines

8.4.1 Colonoscopy Intervals

Colonoscopy is the cornerstone for **colorectal cancer** prevention and early detection:

1. **Average-Risk Individuals**
   - Start at age 45 or 50 (depending on updated guidelines) and repeat every 10 years if normal.
   - Some guidelines recently lowered screening onset to 45 for general population to catch earlier incidence.
2. **Family History**
   - If a first-degree relative had colon cancer or advanced polyps, begin screening earlier (age 40 or 10 years before the affected relative's diagnosis) and repeat more frequently.
3. **IBD Patients**
   - Long-standing ulcerative colitis or Crohn's colitis (8–10 years post-diagnosis) requires more

frequent colonoscopies (every 1–2 years) due to higher cancer risk.

8.4.2 Other Modalities

1. **Flexible Sigmoidoscopy**
   o Screens only the distal colon, typically every 5 years (or combined with yearly fecal occult blood tests). Less common now due to colonoscopy's comprehensiveness.
2. **Fecal Occult Blood Tests (FOBT/FIT)**
   o Annual checking for hidden blood. If positive, colonoscopy indicated.
   o Convenient, non-invasive, but less sensitive for polyps.
3. **CT Colonography**
   o "Virtual colonoscopy" scanning. Good for average-risk screening if colonoscopy is contraindicated, but polyps found still require traditional colonoscopy for removal.
4. **Stool DNA Testing**
   o Cologuard® identifies tumor DNA and occult blood. Positive results necessitate colonoscopy follow-up.

8.5 Higher-Risk Groups

8.5.1 Family History & Genetic Syndromes

1. **Lynch Syndrome (HNPCC)**
   - Autosomal dominant condition with high risk of colon and other cancers (endometrial, stomach).
   - Screening often starts in the 20s or 2–5 years younger than earliest cancer in family.
2. **Familial Adenomatous Polyposis (FAP)**
   - Numerous adenomatous polyps appear in teen years; nearly 100% progression to cancer without colectomy.
   - Requires sigmoidoscopy or colonoscopy screening as early as puberty.

8.5.2 Long-Standing IBD

As mentioned, **ulcerative colitis** or **Crohn's colitis** beyond 8–10 years significantly raises colon cancer risk, justifying more frequent surveillance colonoscopies and biopsies (random or targeted by chromoendoscopy).

8.6 Key Terms Recap

- **Adenomatous Polyp**: Precancerous colon polyp that can progress via the adenoma–carcinoma sequence.
- **Polypectomy**: Removal of polyps during colonoscopy, reducing future cancer risk.

- **Diverticulosis**: Asymptomatic outpouchings in the colon wall; can bleed or become inflamed (diverticulitis).
- **Colonoscopy**: Direct, full visualization of the colon for screening, polyp removal, biopsy.
- **Lynch Syndrome (HNPCC)**: Hereditary colon cancer syndrome with high lifetime risk of various malignancies.
- **FOBT (Fecal Occult Blood Test)**: Annual stool-based screening for hidden blood, a sign of possible colon lesions.

8.7 Quick Quiz

1. **Multiple Choice**: Which polyp type is generally **non-neoplastic** (low malignant potential) unless it meets certain criteria (like sessile serrated features)?
   a) Adenomatous polyp
   b) Hyperplastic polyp
   c) Inflammatory polyp
   d) Villous polyp
2. **True or False**: Diverticulosis often presents with **painless** bleeding or no symptoms at all.
3. **Fill in the Blank**: _____ is commonly recommended as the first-line screening tool for colorectal cancer in average-risk individuals, typically starting at age 45 or 50.

4. **Which syndrome involves numerous adenomatous polyps and near-certain progression to colon cancer by middle age if untreated?**

   a) Peutz–Jeghers syndrome

   b) Familial Adenomatous Polyposis (FAP)

   c) Juvenile polyposis

   d) Lynch syndrome

5. **Short Answer**: Name one reason why individuals with **long-standing ulcerative colitis** require more frequent colonoscopic surveillance than the general population.

Answers

1. **(b) Hyperplastic polyp** – Usually benign but watch for certain serrated subtypes.

2. **True** – Diverticulosis is often asymptomatic or can cause painless rectal bleeding.

3. **Colonoscopy** – The gold standard screening method for colorectal cancer.

4. **(b) Familial Adenomatous Polyposis (FAP)** – Hundreds to thousands of colonic adenomas, nearly 100% cancer risk by 40s if not removed.

5. **Example**: "Long-standing mucosal inflammation elevates cancer risk in UC; frequent colonoscopies detect dysplasia or malignancies early."

Concluding Note

Colorectal diseases range from benign polyps to life-threatening cancers, as well as diverticular complications. Early detection and removal of adenomatous polyps significantly reduce cancer incidence, and screening guidelines—in particular colonoscopy—are paramount. Meanwhile, diverticular disease (diverticulosis or diverticulitis) can remain quiet or flare with inflammation and bleeding. Going forward, Chapter 9 addresses Hepatology: Liver & Biliary Disorders, transitioning our focus from the colon to the liver, gallbladder, and the variety of diseases—viral hepatitis, cirrhosis, gallstones—that can disrupt these essential organs.

Chapter 9: Hepatology — Liver & Biliary Disorders

9.1 The Liver's Essential Functions

9.1.1 Role in Metabolism & Detoxification

The **liver** is a **vital organ** performing numerous critical processes:

1. **Metabolism of Nutrients**
   - Carbohydrates: Stores glycogen, releases glucose (glycogenolysis), synthesizes new glucose (gluconeogenesis).
   - Proteins: Deaminates amino acids, synthesizes plasma proteins (albumin, clotting factors).
   - Fats: Produces bile acids for fat emulsification, packages lipids.
2. **Detoxification**
   - Breaks down or inactivates toxins, drugs, and hormones (e.g., ammonia to urea).
   - Cytochrome P450 enzyme systems within hepatocytes are key here.
3. **Storage**

- Vitamins (A, D, B12) and minerals (iron, copper).
- Releases them as needed to maintain homeostasis.
4. **Immunological**
   - **Kupffer cells** line sinusoids and filter pathogens or debris, complementing overall immune defense.

9.1.2 Bile Production

- **Hepatocytes** produce **bile**, stored in the gallbladder, then released into the duodenum to emulsify dietary fats.
- Waste products like **bilirubin** (from RBC breakdown) are excreted via bile into feces.

9.2 Viral Hepatitis (A, B, C, etc.)

9.2.1 Transmission & Spectrum

Viral hepatitis refers to inflammation of the liver caused by specific viruses labeled **A, B, C, D, E**:

1. **Hepatitis A (HAV)**
   - **Fecal-oral transmission** (contaminated food/water).
   - Usually acute, self-limiting. A vaccine is available.
2. **Hepatitis B (HBV)**

- Blood-borne (sexual contact, IV drug use, perinatal).
- Can be **acute** or become **chronic**, raising the risk for cirrhosis, hepatocellular carcinoma (HCC).
- HBV vaccine part of many national immunization programs.

3. **Hepatitis C (HCV)**
   - Primarily **blood-borne** (shared needles, transfusions before screening).
   - Often **chronic**, leading to progressive liver damage over decades.
   - No current vaccine, but effective **direct-acting antivirals (DAAs)** can achieve cure (sustained virologic response).

4. **Hepatitis D (HDV), E (HEV)**
   - **HDV** requires HBV co-infection.
   - **HEV** typically fecal-oral route in developing regions, can be severe in pregnant women.

9.2.2 Acute vs. Chronic

1. **Acute Hepatitis**
   - Symptoms: Fatigue, anorexia, jaundice, dark urine. Elevated ALT/AST.
   - Usually self-limiting in HAV, HEV; some risk of acute liver failure.

2. **Chronic Hepatitis**
   - Ongoing inflammation beyond **6 months**. Common in HBV, HCV.
   - Gradual scarring → **fibrosis** → possible cirrhosis.
   - Early detection and treatment crucial to prevent advanced disease.

9.2.3 Vaccines & Treatments

1. **Vaccines**
   - **HAV** and **HBV** vaccines recommended in many countries, significantly reducing incidence.
2. **HCV Therapy**
   - Direct-acting antivirals (DAAs) like sofosbuvir/ledipasvir combos can clear the virus in ~95% of chronic HCV patients.
3. **Monitoring**
   - Regular LFTs, viral load tests, screening for HCC in chronic cases.

9.3 Alcoholic & Non-Alcoholic Fatty Liver Disease (NAFLD)

9.3.1 Steatosis, Steatohepatitis (NASH), Cirrhosis

Two major forms of **fatty liver** conditions:

1. **Alcoholic Liver Disease**
   - Chronic alcohol intake → fat accumulation (steatosis) → inflammatory damage (alcoholic hepatitis) → cirrhosis if persistent.
   - Risk correlates with amount/duration of alcohol consumption plus genetic, nutritional, and gender factors.
2. **Non-Alcoholic Fatty Liver Disease (NAFLD)**
   - Often linked to **metabolic syndrome** (obesity, diabetes, dyslipidemia).
   - **NASH (Non-Alcoholic Steatohepatitis)**: The inflammatory subtype that can progress to cirrhosis and HCC.

9.3.2 Progression & Risk Factors

Fatty infiltration by itself (simple steatosis) may not cause severe damage. However, inflammation plus oxidative stress can lead to **fibrosis**:

- **Obesity**, sedentary lifestyles, insulin resistance elevate risk for NAFLD/NASH.
- Genetic predispositions also influence disease severity (e.g., PNPLA3 gene variants).

9.3.3 Lifestyle & Management

1. **Lifestyle Changes**
   - **Weight loss**, dietary improvements (low sugar, low saturated fat), regular exercise.
   - Alcohol cessation for alcoholic steatohepatitis.
2. **Medications**
   - Vitamin E or pioglitazone sometimes tried in NASH.
   - Under investigation: GLP-1 agonists (e.g., semaglutide) for NAFLD associated with T2 diabetes.
3. **Monitoring**
   - Periodic LFTs, imaging (ultrasound, FibroScan), and exclude advanced cirrhosis progression.

9.4 Cirrhosis & Portal Hypertension

9.4.1 Fibrosis Altering Liver Architecture

Cirrhosis is the end stage of **chronic liver disease**, where normal lobular architecture is replaced by **nodules** encased in fibrous bands:

1. **Causes**

- Chronic viral hepatitis (B or C), alcoholic/NASH, autoimmune hepatitis, hemochromatosis, Wilson's disease, etc.

2. **Consequences**
   - **Portal Hypertension**: Elevated pressure in the portal venous system due to increased resistance in the scarred liver.
   - Reduced **synthetic** function (albumin, clotting factors), compromised detox (ammonia buildup).

9.4.2 Complications

1. **Variceal Bleeding**
   - Esophageal or gastric varices can rupture, causing massive hematemesis or melena.
   - **Nonselective β-blockers** (propranolol) or endoscopic banding help prevent bleeds.
2. **Ascites**
   - Fluid accumulation in the peritoneal cavity.
   - Managed with sodium restriction, **diuretics** (spironolactone, furosemide), large-volume paracentesis if refractory.
3. **Hepatic Encephalopathy**
   - Neuropsychiatric manifestations from elevated ammonia, toxins.

o Lactulose and rifaximin used to reduce ammonia absorption.

4. **Hepatorenal Syndrome**

   o Progressive renal failure in advanced cirrhosis.

   o Limited treatment options; poor prognosis without transplant.

9.4.3 Management & TIPS

1. **Medical**

   o Treat underlying etiology (antivirals for hepatitis, abstinence in alcoholic disease).

   o Monitor for varices, ascites, encephalopathy.

2. **TIPS (Transjugular Intrahepatic Portosystemic Shunt)**

   o Creates a channel in the liver parenchyma connecting portal and hepatic veins, reducing portal pressure.

   o Used for recurrent variceal bleeding or difficult ascites but can worsen encephalopathy.

3. **Liver Transplant**

   o Definitive option for end-stage cirrhosis or acute liver failure.

   o Requires thorough pre-transplant evaluation (MELD score) and lifelong immunosuppression.

9.5 Cholestasis & Gallbladder Issues

9.5.1 Gallstones (Cholelithiasis)

Cholelithiasis is the presence of stones (calculi) in the gallbladder, often formed by imbalances in bile components (cholesterol, bilirubin):

1. **Risk Factors** ("5 F's")
   - Female, Fat, Forty, Fertile (multiparity), Fair (in certain epidemiological contexts).
2. **Symptoms**
   - **Biliary colic**: Episodic right upper quadrant (RUQ) or epigastric pain, often postprandial (especially after fatty meals).
   - If a stone obstructs the cystic duct → cholecystitis, causing persistent RUQ pain, fever, leukocytosis.

9.5.2 Cholecystitis & Bile Duct Obstructions

1. **Acute Cholecystitis**
   - Inflammation of the gallbladder, typically from a stone lodged in the cystic duct.
   - RUQ tenderness, positive Murphy's sign, requires antibiotics, possible cholecystectomy.
2. **Choledocholithiasis & Cholangitis**

- Stones in the **common bile duct** → obstructive jaundice, potentially ascending infection (cholangitis) with Charcot's triad (fever, RUQ pain, jaundice).

3. **ERCP (Endoscopic Retrograde Cholangiopancreatography)**
   - Both diagnostic and therapeutic: identifies and removes bile duct stones, places stents if needed.
   - Replaced by MRCP for purely diagnostic imaging in some cases.

9.5.3 Cholestasis

Cholestasis means impaired bile flow:

- **Intrahepatic**: e.g., viral hepatitis, primary biliary cholangitis.
- **Extrahepatic**: e.g., common bile duct stones, strictures, tumors.
- Symptoms: pruritus, jaundice, pale stools, dark urine if bilirubin can't reach the intestine.

9.6 Key Terms Recap

- **Hepatocytes**: Main liver cells performing metabolism, detox, protein synthesis.
- **Cirrhosis**: End-stage fibrosis altering liver structure, leading to portal hypertension and complications.
- **Portal Hypertension**: Elevated portal venous pressure

  → varices, ascites, splenomegaly.
- **NAFLD/NASH**: Metabolic-driven fat accumulation and inflammation in liver, can progress to cirrhosis.
- **Cholelithiasis**: Gallstones in the gallbladder.
- **ERCP**: Procedure to visualize and treat bile duct or pancreatic duct problems (e.g., stone removal).
- **TIPS**: Shunt creation to reduce portal pressure, used in refractory variceal bleeding or ascites.

9.7 Quick Quiz

1. **Multiple Choice**: Which virus typically causes **chronic** hepatitis and has **no** current vaccine, but is curable with modern DAAs?
   a) Hepatitis A
   b) Hepatitis B
   c) Hepatitis C
   d) Hepatitis E
2. **True or False**: NAFLD (non-alcoholic fatty liver disease) can progress to cirrhosis even without any

alcohol intake, especially in the context of obesity or metabolic syndrome.

3. **Fill in the Blank**: _____ is an end-stage pathological condition where normal liver tissue is replaced by regenerative nodules and fibrous bands, often leading to portal hypertension.

4. **Which condition involves inflammation of the gallbladder due to a stone obstructing the cystic duct, typically presenting with RUQ pain and fever?**
   a) Cholelithiasis
   b) Choledocholithiasis
   c) Cholecystitis
   d) Cholangitis

5. **Short Answer**: List two major complications of **portal hypertension** in cirrhosis and explain why they occur.

Answers

1. **(c) Hepatitis C** – No vaccine exists, but curable with direct-acting antivirals.

2. **True** – NAFLD can indeed lead to cirrhosis, especially with NASH.

3. **Cirrhosis** – Irreversible liver scarring and nodular regeneration.

4. **(c) Cholecystitis** – Stone obstructs the cystic duct, leading to inflammation, pain, fever.

5. **Example**: "Variceal bleeding (due to high portal pressure in esophageal/gastric collaterals) and ascites (because portal hypertension + hypoalbuminemia fosters fluid leakage into the peritoneal space)."

Final Thoughts

Hepatology underscores the **liver's essential functions**—from detoxification to nutrient metabolism—and how **chronic insults** (viruses, fat accumulation, alcohol) can reshape this vital organ into **cirrhosis** with severe clinical ramifications. Meanwhile, the **biliary system** can give rise to painful or life-threatening episodes when obstructed by gallstones. In **Chapter 10**, we'll shift toward **pancreatic conditions**, exploring acute and chronic pancreatitis plus the complexities of **pancreatic cancer**, further illustrating how interconnected and critical each accessory organ is to overall digestive health.

Chapter 10: Pancreatic Conditions

10.1 The Pancreas: A Dual-Function Organ

10.1.1 Exocrine vs. Endocrine Roles

The **pancreas** lies behind the stomach, stretching across the back of the abdomen. It serves:

1. **Exocrine Function**
   - **Acinar cells** produce digestive enzymes (amylase, lipase, proteases) secreted into the duodenum.
   - **Bicarbonate** from ductal cells neutralizes gastric acid, ensuring optimal pH for enzyme activity.
2. **Endocrine Function**
   - **Islets of Langerhans** secrete hormones, chiefly **insulin** (lowers blood glucose) and **glucagon** (raises blood glucose).
   - Balance of these hormones is vital for metabolic homeostasis; disruptions can cause diabetes mellitus.

A myriad of conditions can compromise these roles, leading to maldigestion (exocrine failure) or metabolic disorders (endocrine failure), as seen in chronic pancreatitis or advanced disease.

10.2 Acute Pancreatitis

10.2.1 Common Triggers

Acute pancreatitis is sudden, often severe, inflammation of the pancreas:

1. **Gallstones (Cholelithiasis)**
   - A stone migrating into the common bile duct can obstruct the pancreatic duct.
   - Bile reflux or ductal hypertension inflames the pancreatic tissue.
2. **Alcohol Use**
   - Chronic or binge drinking can injure acinar cells, predispose to enzyme activation within the gland.
   - Accounts for a large fraction of acute pancreatitis cases in many regions.
3. **Hypertriglyceridemia**
   - Extremely high triglyceride levels (>1000 mg/dL) can precipitate acute pancreatitis.
   - Other triggers: Medications, trauma, infections, ERCP complications.

10.2.2 Clinical Features

1. **Epigastric Pain**
   - Often **severe**, boring pain radiating to the back, possibly improved by leaning forward.
   - Nausea, vomiting frequently accompany it.
2. **Elevated Amylase/Lipase**
   - At least **3× the upper limit** is highly suggestive. **Lipase** is more specific to the pancreas.
   - Imaging (CT scan, ultrasound) can confirm severity or reveal complications (necrosis, pseudocyst).
3. **Complications**
   - **Hypovolemia**: Fluid shifts into inflamed pancreatic bed.
   - **Necrotizing Pancreatitis**: Risk of infection in necrotic tissue.
   - **Organ Failure** (respiratory, renal) if severe.

10.2.3 Supportive Therapy & Management

1. **Fluid Resuscitation**
   - Large volumes of IV fluids to maintain perfusion, correct intravascular depletion.
2. **Pain Control**
   - IV opioids (e.g., fentanyl) or patient-controlled analgesia.

3. **Nutritional Support**
   - Mild cases: Oral feeding can resume when tolerated.
   - Severe: May require enteral feeding via nasojejunal tube to "rest" the pancreas while still providing gut nutrition.
4. **Gallstone-Related**
   - ERCP if cholangitis or persistent obstruction.
   - Cholecystectomy once inflammation subsides to prevent recurrence.

10.3 Chronic Pancreatitis

10.3.1 Progressive Damage & Scarring

Chronic pancreatitis involves **repeated** or **ongoing** pancreatic injury, leading to fibrotic changes and permanent dysfunction:

1. **Etiologies**
   - Long-term alcohol abuse (most common in adults).
   - Genetic causes (hereditary pancreatitis), autoimmune pancreatitis, or consequence of severe acute episodes.
2. **Pathophysiology**

- Inflammation → scarring → loss of acinar cells and ductal patency.
- Eventually, both **exocrine** (enzyme) and **endocrine** (insulin) functions can fail.

10.3.2 Clinical Manifestations

1. **Chronic Epigastric Pain**
   - Recurrent or persistent, may radiate to the back.
   - Food intake often triggers pain, resulting in weight loss from fear of eating.
2. **Malabsorption & Steatorrhea**
   - Insufficient pancreatic enzymes cause **fat malabsorption**, leading to greasy, foul-smelling stools.
   - Vitamin deficiencies (A, D, E, K) can occur.
3. **Diabetes Mellitus**
   - Loss of insulin-producing islet cells → "Type 3c diabetes."
   - May be brittle and hard to control due to concurrent glucagon deficiency.

10.3.3 Pain Control & Enzyme Replacement

1. **Pain Management**

- NSAIDs, acetaminophen, or opioids (in severe cases).
- Adjuvant therapies (pregabalin) for neuropathic pain.

2. **Pancreatic Enzyme Replacement**
   - **Pancrelipase** (lipase, amylase, protease) improves nutrient absorption, reduces steatorrhea.
   - Taken with meals to augment digestion.

3. **Endoscopic or Surgical Interventions**
   - Drain pseudocysts if symptomatic.
   - Decompress obstructed ducts or remove severely damaged pancreatic tissue in advanced cases.

10.4 Pancreatic Cancer

10.4.1 Risk Factors & Presentation

Pancreatic adenocarcinoma (exocrine) is notorious for late detection and poor prognosis:

1. **Risk Factors**
   - Chronic pancreatitis (especially hereditary), **smoking**, long-standing diabetes, obesity, certain genetic syndromes (BRCA2 mutations).

2. **Clinical Clues**
   - **Painless jaundice** if tumor blocks the common bile duct (head of pancreas).
   - Weight loss, vague upper abdominal/back pain.
   - New-onset or poorly controlled diabetes in older adults might hint at an occult tumor.

10.4.2 Diagnosis & Poor Prognosis

1. **Imaging**
   - **CT scan** with pancreatic protocol identifies masses, vascular involvement, metastasis.
   - Endoscopic ultrasound (EUS) for fine-needle aspiration biopsies.
2. **Tumor Markers**
   - **CA 19-9** can be elevated but lacks specificity.
3. **Prognosis**
   - Typically discovered at advanced stages, 5-year survival remains low (~10% overall).
   - Early detection is key but uncommon.

10.4.3 Whipple Procedure & Supportive Care

1. **Whipple Procedure (Pancreaticoduodenectomy)**
   - For resectable tumors in the pancreatic head. Removes the head of the pancreas, duodenum, part of bile duct, gallbladder.

- Challenging surgery with potential complications (fistulas, delayed gastric emptying).
2. **Adjuvant Therapy**
   - **Chemotherapy** (gemcitabine, FOLFIRINOX) and/or radiation for local–regional control.
3. **Palliative Measures**
   - Pain management, stenting for biliary obstruction, nutritional support.
   - Patients with advanced disease often benefit from hospice involvement for quality-of-life improvements.

10.5 Key Terms Recap

- **Amylase & Lipase**: Digestive enzymes, elevated in pancreatitis (lipase more pancreas-specific).
- **Steatorrhea**: Fat-laden stools due to inadequate pancreatic lipase.
- **Pancreatic Enzyme Replacement**: Oral capsules (e.g., pancrelipase) aiding digestion in chronic pancreatitis or post-pancreatectomy.
- **Whipple Procedure**: Surgical resection for pancreatic head tumors, involving pancreaticoduodenectomy.
- **Pancreatic Adenocarcinoma**: Highly lethal cancer, often silent until advanced stages, requiring complex multimodal treatment.

10.6 Quick Quiz

1. **Multiple Choice**: Which two factors are **most commonly** implicated in acute pancreatitis?

    a) Hypercalcemia and celiac disease

    b) Gallstones and alcohol abuse

    c) Low-protein diet and osteoporosis

    d) Trauma and IBS

2. **True or False**: Chronic pancreatitis frequently leads to **diabetes mellitus** due to loss of insulin-producing cells.

3. **Fill in the Blank**: Patients with chronic pancreatitis may develop **steatorrhea** because of insufficient _____ secretion, limiting fat digestion.

4. **Which procedure is used to remove the head of the pancreas, duodenum, gallbladder, and part of the bile duct in select cases of resectable pancreatic cancer?**

    a) TIPS

    b) Cholecystectomy

    c) Whipple procedure (pancreaticoduodenectomy)

    d) Subtotal colectomy

5. **Short Answer**: Why does **pancreatic cancer** typically present with a poor prognosis?

Answers

1. **(b) Gallstones and alcohol abuse** – The two most frequent triggers of acute pancreatitis.
2. **True** – Chronic inflammation and scarring can destroy islet cells, prompting secondary (Type 3c) diabetes.
3. **Pancreatic enzymes (e.g., lipase)** – Without adequate lipase, dietary fats aren't broken down.
4. **(c) Whipple procedure (pancreaticoduodenectomy)** – Standard surgical approach for tumors in the pancreatic head.
5. **Example**: "It's often asymptomatic or nonspecific in early stages, leading to late diagnosis when cancer is already locally advanced or metastatic."

Concluding Note

Acute pancreatitis is a painful, acute inflammation commonly linked to gallstones or alcohol, while **chronic pancreatitis** gradually destroys pancreatic tissue, causing **malabsorption** and frequent pain. **Pancreatic cancer**, one of the deadliest malignancies, underscores the **importance of early detection**—though that remains challenging. In **Chapter 11**, we'll transition to **GI Infections & Parasites**, reviewing how pathogens can cause diarrheal illnesses, colitis, or more systemic complications, further illustrating how varied the scope of GI health can be.

Chapter 11: GI Infections & Parasites

11.1 Common Infectious Diarrhea

11.1.1 Bacterial & Viral Causes

Acute infectious diarrhea is a leading cause of morbidity worldwide, varying by pathogen and severity:

1. **Bacterial Pathogens**
    o   **Salmonella**: Often from poultry, eggs; causes gastroenteritis with fever, sometimes invasive in immunocompromised.
    o   **Shigella**: Transmitted via fecal-oral route (contaminated water/food), can be invasive, leading to dysentery (bloody diarrhea).
    o   **Enterotoxigenic E. coli (ETEC)**: "Traveler's diarrhea," watery stools, abdominal cramping.
    o   **Campylobacter jejuni**: Common in poultry, can cause severe inflammatory diarrhea, possible complication: Guillain–Barré syndrome.
2. **Viral Pathogens**

- Norovirus: Highly contagious, outbreak-prone in cruise ships, schools; abrupt onset vomiting/diarrhea, resolves quickly.
- Rotavirus: Leading cause of infantile diarrhea in unvaccinated populations; rotavirus vaccine has reduced prevalence.
- Adenovirus, Astrovirus: Additional viral causes of mild GI upset.

11.1.2 Clinical Management

1. **Fluid Rehydration**
   - Mainstay to avoid dehydration (oral rehydration salts or IV fluids in severe cases).
   - Electrolyte replacement if losses are profound.
2. **Antibiotics**
   - Indicated for **severe** bacterial infections, invasive organisms (Shigella, some Salmonella) or high-risk patients (immunocompromised).
   - Overuse can disrupt normal flora, potentially leading to **C. difficile** overgrowth.
3. **Supportive Therapy**
   - Antimotility agents (e.g., loperamide) may reduce symptoms in noninvasive diarrhea but should be avoided if invasive/bloody diarrhea is suspected.
4. **Prevention**

- Handwashing, proper food handling, traveler's caution with local water/food sources, vaccines (e.g., rotavirus, cholera, typhoid in endemic areas).

11.2 Clostridioides difficile (C. diff) Infection

11.2.1 Antibiotic-Associated Colitis

Clostridioides difficile, a spore-forming bacterium, flourishes when normal gut flora is disturbed—**often by broad-spectrum antibiotics**:

1. **Toxins**
   - TcdA (toxin A) and TcdB (toxin B) cause mucosal injury, inflammation, and diarrhea.
   - Ranges from mild colitis to severe pseudomembranous colitis.
2. **Risk Factors**
   - Recent hospitalization, antibiotic use (fluoroquinolones, cephalosporins, clindamycin).
   - Advanced age, immunocompromise, prolonged hospital stays.

11.2.2 Diagnosis & Treatment

1. **Diagnostic Tests**
   - **Stool PCR** for C. diff toxin genes or **enzyme immunoassays** for toxins.
   - GDH (glutamate dehydrogenase) + toxin assay or two-step algorithm confirm active infection.
2. **Therapeutic Agents**
   - **Oral vancomycin** or **fidaxomicin** are first-line for initial or recurrent infections.
   - Metronidazole is less favored now except in mild cases when others are unavailable.
3. **Fecal Microbiota Transplant (FMT)**
   - **Refractory or recurrent** cases often respond to transplanted stool from healthy donors, restoring normal microbiota.
   - Administered via colonoscopy, enema, or naso-enteric tube; high success rates.

11.2.3 Infection Control

- **Contact Precautions**: Proper hand hygiene (soap, not just sanitizer, as spores resist alcohol), isolation of infected patients.
- **Antibiotic Stewardship**: Judicious prescribing reduces risk by maintaining gut flora balance.

11.3 Traveler's Diarrhea

11.3.1 Epidemiology & Causes

Traveler's diarrhea commonly strikes visitors to regions with suboptimal water treatment or hygiene practices:

- **ETEC (Enterotoxigenic E. coli)**: Leading cause, producing toxins that cause watery diarrhea.
- Other suspects: Shigella, Campylobacter, protozoa (Giardia) in some areas.

11.3.2 Prophylactic Measures

1. **Safe Drinking Water**
   - Boiling, filtering, or using bottled water. Avoid ice made from tap water.
2. **Food Precautions**
   - No raw/undercooked meats, unpasteurized dairy, or produce that can't be peeled.
3. **Vaccinations**
   - Hepatitis A, typhoid vaccine recommended for certain travel destinations.
4. **Prophylactic Antibiotics**
   - Short-term use in high-risk travelers or critical schedules, though not universally recommended to avoid resistance.

11.3.3 Management

- **Rehydration** remains core therapy.
- **Antimotility** agents can reduce frequency.
- **Empirical antibiotics** (e.g., fluoroquinolones, azithromycin, rifaximin) if moderate-severe or persists > 2 days.

11.4 Parasitic Infestations

11.4.1 Giardia lamblia

Giardiasis is a protozoan infection from **contaminated water** (mountain streams, daycare centers):

1. **Pathophysiology**
   - Trophozoites colonize the small intestine, interfering with fat absorption → **greasy stools**.
2. **Symptoms**
   - Bloating, flatulence, foul-smelling diarrhea, malabsorption (steatorrhea).
3. **Diagnosis & Treatment**
   - Stool O&P (ova & parasites) or antigen tests.
   - **Metronidazole** or **tinidazole** typically effective.

11.4.2 Entamoeba histolytica

Amebiasis results from ingestion of cysts in contaminated food/water:

1. **Invasive Dysentery**
   - Abdominal pain, bloody diarrhea, possible extraintestinal spread (liver abscess).
2. **Diagnostics**
   - Stool microscopy (O&P), antigen testing, serology.
3. **Therapy**
   - Metronidazole or tinidazole for invasive disease, followed by a luminal agent (paromomycin) to clear intraluminal cysts.

11.4.3 Helminths (Worms)

Helminthic infections (roundworms, tapeworms, flukes):

- **Ascaris lumbricoides** (roundworm) can cause intestinal or lung migration.

- **Hookworms** lead to chronic blood loss → anemia.

- **Tapeworms** like Taenia solium can cause cysticercosis if eggs invade tissues.

- Management: antihelminthic drugs (albendazole, mebendazole, praziquantel) depending on worm type.

11.5 Key Terms Recap

- **C. difficile**: Antibiotic-associated colitis agent, producing toxins; treat with oral vancomycin or fidaxomicin.
- **Traveler's Diarrhea**: Typically watery diarrhea from ETEC; prophylaxis includes careful food/water precautions.
- **Giardia lamblia**: Protozoan causing malabsorptive diarrhea (steatorrhea), "camping diarrhea."
- **Fecal O&P**: Standard stool test for ova and parasites diagnosing amebiasis, giardiasis, etc.
- **Rehydration**: Foundational therapy for most diarrheal illnesses to prevent dehydration.

11.6 Quick Quiz

1. **Multiple Choice**: Which pathogen is most commonly linked to **antibiotic-associated colitis** and pseudomembranous colitis?
   a) Salmonella enteritidis
   b) Norovirus
   c) Clostridioides difficile
   d) Giardia lamblia
2. **True or False**: The first-line treatment for severe or recurrent C. diff infections is oral **metronidazole**.

3. **Fill in the Blank**: _____ is a protozoan commonly found in contaminated water, leading to foul-smelling, greasy stools and malabsorption symptoms.

4. **Which strategy is not recommended for preventing traveler's diarrhea?**

   a) Avoid drinking tap water or using ice made from it

   b) Vaccinate against hepatitis A

   c) Drinking bottled carbonated beverages freely

   d) Routinely using high-dose antibiotics for everyone traveling

5. **Short Answer**: Give one example of a viral cause of acute gastroenteritis, along with its typical mode of transmission.

Answers

1. **(c) Clostridioides difficile** – Key culprit in antibiotic-associated colitis.

2. **False** – Oral **vancomycin** or **fidaxomicin** is now preferred; metronidazole is second-line or reserved for mild cases if others are unavailable.

3. **Giardia lamblia** – The leading cause of camping-related protozoal infections.

4. **(d) Routinely using high-dose antibiotics for everyone traveling** – Overuse fosters resistance and

side effects; prophylaxis is considered only for specific high-risk groups.

5. **Example**: "Norovirus often spreads via contaminated food, water, or close contact, frequently causing outbreaks on cruise ships or in communal settings."

Concluding Note

GI infections range from acute, self-limiting diarrheas to more severe or recurrent diseases (like **C. difficile** or **amebiasis**). Proper **identification** of the pathogen (via stool tests, history of travel, antibiotic exposure) and **targeted treatment** (rehydration, appropriate antimicrobials) are crucial for full recovery. In the next chapter (**Chapter 12**), we'll explore **Pediatric Gastroenterology Essentials**, highlighting unique GI conditions and considerations for infants and children, further expanding our comprehension of digestive health across age groups.

Chapter 12: Pediatric Gastroenterology Essentials

12.1 How Pediatric GI Differs from Adult GI

1. **Anatomical & Physiological Variations**
   - Smaller stomach capacity, faster gastric emptying (in younger infants), intestinal enzyme levels still maturing.
   - Different microbiome composition early in life; breastfed vs. formula-fed differences.
2. **Developmental Considerations**
   - Infant feeding transitions: breast milk or formula, introduction of solids around 4–6 months.
   - Toilet training, picky eaters, and rapid growth spurts can all impact GI health.

Throughout infancy and childhood, growth and development interplay with GI function, shaping nutritional requirements and susceptibilities to certain disorders.

12.2 Reflux in Infants

12.2.1 Physiologic vs. GERD

Infant reflux is remarkably common due to shorter esophagus, lower esophageal sphincter immaturity, and frequent liquid feeding:

1. **Physiologic Reflux (Spitting Up)**
   - Occurs in many healthy infants, peaks at 3–4 months, improving by 1 year.
   - Generally not concerning if the infant is gaining weight well and has no respiratory or feeding issues.

2. **GERD (Gastroesophageal Reflux Disease)**
   - Diagnosed when **reflux** leads to troubling symptoms (e.g., failure to thrive, irritability, recurrent wheezing, feeding aversion).
   - Alarm features: significant discomfort, persistent cough, aspiration pneumonia, weight faltering.

12.2.2 Red Flags & Management

1. **Failure to Thrive**
   - A child dropping in percentiles of weight or height growth can indicate reflux severity or an alternative pathology.

2. **Respiratory Issues**
   - Chronic cough, recurrent pneumonia, or apnea spells raise concern.
3. **Treatment Strategies**
   - **Positioning**: Keeping the infant upright after feeding, slight incline for sleep (while following safe-sleep guidelines).
   - **Feed Adjustments**: Smaller, more frequent feeds, thickened feeds if recommended.
   - **Medications**: Acid-suppressive therapy (H2 blockers or PPIs) if symptoms are severe.
   - **Surgery (Fundoplication)**: Rarely needed except in severe, resistant GERD.

12.3 Common Malabsorption in Children

12.3.1 Cow's Milk Protein Allergy

1. **Pathophysiology**
   - Immune-mediated reaction to proteins in cow's milk (casein, whey).
   - Typically presents in infancy—formula-fed or if dairy in maternal diet passes through breast milk.
2. **Symptoms**

- Diarrhea, vomiting, eczema, colic-like irritability, sometimes bloody stools.
- Failure to thrive in more severe cases.

3. **Management**
   - **Elimination Diet**: Extensively hydrolyzed or amino acid-based formulas.
   - **Breastfeeding Mothers**: Removal of dairy from maternal diet, ensuring adequate calcium/vitamin D from other sources.

12.3.2 Celiac Disease in Children

1. **Presentation**
   - Similar to adults: diarrhea, bloating, irritability, poor growth, and delayed puberty if severe.
   - More subtle signs: enamel defects, recurrent abdominal pain, or mild anemia.

2. **Diagnosis**
   - **tTG-IgA** test (check total IgA to avoid false negatives).
   - Duodenal biopsy for confirmation.

3. **Treatment**
   - **Strict gluten-free diet**; improved growth and symptom resolution typically seen.

12.3.3 Nutritional Deficits

- Children have higher **per-kg nutrient demands**, so malabsorption can rapidly cause **growth delays**.
- **Iron deficiency**, vitamin D deficiency, and others can result in stunted growth or rickets.

12.4 Constipation & Encopresis

12.4.1 Functional vs. Organic Causes

Functional constipation is frequently seen in pediatrics, often during **toilet training** phases or after a painful stool episode:

1. **Functional**
   - No anatomical abnormality; might stem from **withholding behaviors** (fear of painful defecation).
   - Hard, infrequent stools, sometimes resulting in overflow soiling (encopresis).
2. **Organic**
   - Check for hypothyroidism, Hirschsprung disease, spinal abnormalities, or celiac disease if red flags exist (e.g., poor growth, severe abdominal distension).

12.4.2 Toilet Training & Strategies

1. **Toilet Training**

- Gentle approach, avoiding pressure or negative reinforcement.
- Regular "toilet sitting" times after meals to sync with gastrocolic reflex.

2. **Diet & Hydration**
   - Adequate fiber for age, sufficient fluid intake.
3. **Medications**
   - **Osmotic Laxatives** (polyethylene glycol) or stool softeners often first-line.
   - **Behavioral Therapy** if withholding is emotionally/behaviorally driven.

12.5 Colic & Abdominal Pain

12.5.1 Infant Colic

Colic commonly describes episodes of **excessive, unexplained crying** in infants younger than ~4 months:

1. **Rule of Threes**
   - Crying >3 hours/day, >3 days/week, >3 weeks in an otherwise healthy infant.
2. **Potential Causes**
   - Overstimulation, immature nervous system, possible gut discomfort (gas).

- No definitive single cause identified; many theories exist.

12.5.2 Soothing & When to Suspect Pathology

1. **Soothing Techniques**
   - Swaddling, gentle rocking, white noise, pacifiers, trial of maternal diet adjustments if suspecting cow's milk protein sensitivity.
2. **Red Flags**
   - Poor feeding, blood in stool, persistent vomiting, fever, abnormal growth parameters—these suggest an underlying organic disease.
3. **Feeding Techniques**
   - Ensuring proper latch or bottle angle to minimize air swallowing.
   - Burping the infant thoroughly post-feed.

12.6 Key Terms Recap

- **GERD in Infants**: Reflux that causes troublesome symptoms (weight loss, respiratory issues).
- **Cow's Milk Protein Allergy**: Immune reaction to cow's milk proteins, often causing colic, bloody stools, or eczema in young infants.

- **Encopresis**: Fecal incontinence often due to chronic constipation and overflow.
- **Colic**: Excessive infant crying without a clear medical cause, typically resolving by 3–4 months of age.

12.7 Quick Quiz

1. **Multiple Choice**: Which of the following is **not** typically a "red flag" for pathological infant reflux (as opposed to physiologic spit-up)?
   a) Failure to thrive
   b) Post-feeding irritability but no other issues
   c) Recurrent pneumonia
   d) Significant hematemesis
2. **True or False**: Cow's milk protein allergy always presents with severe bloody diarrhea and failure to thrive.
3. **Fill in the Blank**: A child with **constipation** who withholds stools can develop _____, where partially liquid stool leaks around an impaction, leading to soiling.
4. **Which condition is defined by excessive, unexplained infant crying for more than 3 hours a day, at least 3 days a week, in an otherwise healthy infant?**
   a) GERD

b) Colic

c) Failure to thrive

d) Encopresis

5. **Short Answer**: Provide one strategy to manage functional constipation in a preschool-aged child and explain why it helps.

Answers

1. **(b) Post-feeding irritability but no other issues** – Might still be normal spitting up. FTT, recurrent pneumonia, or GI bleeding are more serious signals.

2. **False** – Some present subtly, e.g., mild colic or rash. Not all are severely symptomatic.

3. **Encopresis** – The term describing stool soiling due to chronic withholding and overflow.

4. **(b) Colic** – Excessive crying without an obvious cause.

5. **Example**: "Scheduling regular toilet times after meals helps harness the gastrocolic reflex and fosters consistent bowel movements, reducing stool withholding."

Concluding Perspective

Pediatric gastroenterology accounts for developmental nuances, higher nutrient demands, and unique feeding/behavioral milestones. **Infant reflux** is often benign but can cross into pathologic GERD if it hinders growth or causes respiratory issues. **Malabsorption** (milk protein allergy, celiac), **constipation**, and **colic** can each disrupt family life if not properly addressed, yet in most cases, modifications in diet, behavior, or mild medical interventions bring relief. In **Chapter 13**, we'll turn to **Lifestyle & Preventive Strategies** for broader GI health—covering the value of proper nutrition, exercise, and screening in preventing digestive troubles across all ages.

Chapter 13: Lifestyle & Preventive Strategies

13.1 Diet & Nutrition for GI Health

13.1.1 Balanced Fiber Intake

1. **Soluble vs. Insoluble Fiber**
   - **Soluble fiber** (oats, beans, psyllium) forms a gel-like substance, slowing digestion and aiding in cholesterol management.
   - **Insoluble fiber** (wheat bran, vegetables) adds bulk, promoting regular bowel movements and preventing constipation.
   - **Combining both types** helps maintain healthy digestion, though certain GI conditions (like IBS) may need individualized approaches (e.g., low-FODMAP to reduce bloating).

2. **Probiotic & Fermented Foods**
   - Yogurt, kefir, sauerkraut, kimchi, and probiotic supplements can bolster gut microbiome diversity.

- A healthy microbiome can reduce inflammation, support immune function, and stabilize bowel habits (less diarrhea/constipation).

3. **Hydration**
   - Adequate fluid intake assists fiber in moving contents smoothly through the bowel.
   - Dehydration can harden stools, increasing constipation risk.

13.1.2 Minimizing Processed Items & Alcohol

1. **Processed Foods & Fad Diets**
   - Ultra-processed products often contain high sugar, salt, saturated fats—promoting obesity, non-alcoholic fatty liver disease (NAFLD).
   - Restrictive fad diets may lead to deficiencies (vitamins, minerals) if prolonged or done without supervision.

2. **Alcohol Moderation**
   - Excessive alcohol intake is a leading cause of **alcoholic liver disease** and acute pancreatitis.
   - Moderation guidelines generally limit men to ≤2 drinks/day, women ≤1 drink/day (U.S. standards), though less is preferable for optimal GI health.

13.2 Exercise & Stress Reduction

13.2.1 Lowering GI-Related Risks

1. **Obesity Prevention**
   - Regular physical activity helps manage body weight, diminishing risk of GERD, gallstones, and NAFLD.
   - Enhanced insulin sensitivity reduces metabolic syndrome components that affect GI health (e.g., hyperlipidemia → pancreatitis risk).

2. **Improved Motility**
   - Exercise stimulates the gastrocolic reflex, promoting regular bowel movements.
   - Studies suggest moderate activity decreases chances of constipation and diverticular complications.

13.2.2 Stress & Mental Well-Being

1. **Brain–Gut Axis**
   - Chronic stress can exacerbate functional GI disorders like IBS, cause or worsen reflux episodes, or hamper IBD control.

- ○ Cortisol and other stress hormones may alter gut motility and microbiome composition.
2. **Mindful Techniques & Therapies**
   - ○ **Yoga, meditation, cognitive behavioral therapy (CBT)** can reduce perceived pain, regulate motility, and calm GI upset.
   - ○ Stress management is a key element in comprehensive GI care—particularly for functional syndromes.

13.3 Screening & Early Detection

13.3.1 Colonoscopy & Other Tests

1. **Colonoscopy**
   - ○ Gold standard for **colon polyp** detection and **colorectal cancer** screening; recommended starting age ~45 or 50 for average-risk individuals (guidelines vary).
   - ○ Frequency depends on polyp findings, family history, or other risk factors.
2. **Risk-Based Endoscopic Surveillance**
   - ○ **Barrett's esophagus**: Regular EGD to catch dysplasia early.
   - ○ **H. pylori Testing**: Non-invasive breath/stool tests or endoscopic biopsy in dyspepsia and high-

prevalence areas, helps prevent peptic ulcers and gastric cancer.

3. **Family or Personal History**

 o Inflammatory bowel disease (IBD) involving the colon → more frequent colonoscopies after 8–10 years.

 o Genetic syndromes (Lynch, FAP) → earlier/more frequent colon exams.

13.3.2 Blood & Stool Screening

* **FOBT/FIT (Fecal Occult Blood / Fecal Immunochemical Test)**: Annual checks can detect hidden bleeding, prompting colonoscopy if positive.
* **Serologic Markers**: Rarely used as primary screening but helpful in suspicion of celiac (tTG-IgA) or hepatitis viruses.

13.4 Avoiding Toxins & Excess

13.4.1 Alcohol & Substance Use

Excess alcohol, as noted, leads to:

- **Alcoholic steatohepatitis** (fatty liver, cirrhosis).
- **Acute pancreatitis** due to direct acinar cell damage.
- **Esophageal varices** secondary to cirrhosis, risking life-threatening bleeds.

13.4.2 Mindful Use of NSAIDs

NSAIDs (ibuprofen, naproxen) can cause **peptic ulcers**, GI bleeding, and hamper kidney function, especially when overused:

- **Alternatives**: Acetaminophen for mild pain if no liver damage, or short NSAID courses if needed.
- **Gastroprotection**: If NSAIDs required long-term, PPIs or misoprostol might protect the stomach.

13.4.3 Curbing High-Sugar Diets

High-fructose/sugar diets contribute to **obesity**, fueling NAFLD, metabolic syndrome, and insulin resistance:

- Replacing sweetened beverages with water or unsweetened tea helps maintain normal body weight, reduce the risk of gallstones, and lessen reflux triggers.

13.5 Immunizations

13.5.1 Hepatitis A & B Vaccines

1. **Hepatitis A (HAV)**
   - Fecal-oral transmission; typically mild but can be severe in adults.
   - Vaccination recommended in childhood or before travel to endemic areas.
2. **Hepatitis B (HBV)**
   - Blood-borne or sexual transmission; high risk of chronic infection leading to cirrhosis, hepatocellular carcinoma.
   - **HBV vaccine** part of many national immunization schedules, crucial in infancy.

13.5.2 Rotavirus Vaccine in Infants

Rotavirus is a common cause of severe diarrhea in young children:

- **Oral vaccines** significantly reduce hospitalizations and mortality from rotavirus gastroenteritis.
- Typically administered in early infancy (2-4-6 months, depending on regimen).

13.5.3 Other Pertinent Vaccines

- **Influenza**: Minimizes respiratory or extra GI complications that could flare existing GI disorders.
- **Typhoid**: For travelers to high-risk regions.
- **COVID-19**: Reduces severe infection, which can impact GI tracts secondarily.

13.6 Key Terms Recap

- **Low-FODMAP Diet**: Approach limiting fermentable carbs to ease IBS symptoms.
- **H. pylori Testing**: Checking for stomach bacterium causing ulcers, recommended in dyspepsia or high-prevalence areas.
- **FOBT/FIT**: Stool tests for hidden blood, indicative of possible polyps or colon cancer.
- **NSAID**: Common pain relievers potentially causing peptic ulcers with overuse or poor GI protection.
- **Rotavirus Vaccine**: Prevents severe infantile diarrhea.

13.7 Quick Quiz

1. **Multiple Choice**: Which lifestyle factor is **most** clearly linked to reducing the incidence of non-alcoholic fatty liver disease (NAFLD)?
   a) High-protein diet
   b) Regular exercise and weight control

c) Over-the-counter probiotics

d) High-fat meals at regular intervals

2. **True or False**: Routine colonoscopy screening can effectively prevent many cases of colon cancer by detecting and removing precancerous polyps.

3. **Fill in the Blank**: **NSAIDs** can cause gastric **ulcers** and GI bleeding if used excessively or without proper _____ (e.g., PPI co-therapy in high-risk individuals).

4. **Which childhood vaccine significantly decreases the rate of severe diarrheal disease caused by a viral pathogen?**

a) Hepatitis B vaccine

b) DTaP vaccine

c) Rotavirus vaccine

d) HPV vaccine

5. **Short Answer**: Name one practical strategy for maintaining a balanced gut microbiome and explain its benefit.

Answers

1. **(b) Regular exercise and weight control** – Key to minimizing NAFLD progression.

2. **True** – Colonoscopy can find and remove adenomas, blocking progression to malignant lesions.

3. **Gastroprotection** or "protection" – PPI or misoprostol may protect the gastric mucosa.
4. **(c) Rotavirus vaccine** – Reduces infant diarrhea incidence.
5. **Example**: "Consuming fermented foods (yogurt, kefir) can introduce beneficial bacteria that support gut health, reducing inflammation and improving digestion."

Final Thoughts

Healthy **lifestyle** habits—optimal nutrition, exercise, stress management, and prudent medical screenings—lay the foundation for robust GI health at every age. From **weight management** countering NAFLD to **immunizations** fending off infectious causes of hepatitis or rotavirus diarrhea, prevention is often more powerful (and less costly) than cure. In the next and **final Chapter 14** (*FAQs & Common Myths in Gastroenterology*), we'll tackle widespread misconceptions—from "spicy foods always cause ulcers" to "colonoscopies are only for the elderly"—cementing your grasp of how to keep the digestive system in top shape.

Chapter 14: FAQs & Common Myths in Gastroenterology

14.1 Myths vs. Facts

14.1.1 "Spicy Foods Always Cause Ulcers."

- **Myth**: Many believe that eating spicy dishes leads to **peptic ulcers**.
- **Fact**: While spicy meals may **irritate** an existing ulcer or inflame gastritis symptoms, they **don't typically create ulcers** on their own. The main culprits of peptic ulcers include **Helicobacter pylori** infection and **NSAID overuse**.
- **Takeaway**: Moderation in spicy foods can reduce discomfort if you already have reflux or gastritis, but they're not the primary cause of ulcers.

14.1.2 "Celiac Disease Is Just a Fad."

- **Myth**: Some dismiss celiac as a trendy "gluten-free" hype.

- **Fact**: **Celiac disease** is an **autoimmune disorder**, causing **villous atrophy** and real malabsorption if gluten is consumed. Removing gluten halts the immune-mediated damage and alleviates symptoms.
- **Takeaway**: While not everyone who avoids gluten is celiac, for those diagnosed, a strict gluten-free diet is medically essential, not optional.

14.1.3 "You Can't Have IBS If Your Colonoscopy Is Normal."

- **Myth**: People assume normal imaging/colonoscopy rules out GI pathology.
- **Fact**: **Irritable Bowel Syndrome (IBS)** is a **functional** disorder, meaning routine tests (colonoscopy, imaging) often appear normal. Diagnosis relies on the **Rome IV criteria** and symptom patterns, not visible inflammation or lesions.
- **Takeaway**: Normal scope findings actually *support* the IBS diagnosis when alarm features are excluded.

14.1.4 "All Ulcers Come From Stress Alone."

- **Myth**: Stress can exacerbate stomach issues, but it's not the main underlying factor.
- **Fact**: **Helicobacter pylori** infection and **NSAIDs** remain the primary causes of **peptic ulcers**. Psychological

stress may aggravate symptoms or hamper healing, yet it isn't the sole culprit.

- **Takeaway**: Addressing infection (H. pylori eradication) or protective medication while on NSAIDs is crucial. Reducing stress helps symptom relief but rarely cures ulcers on its own.

14.1.5 "Colonoscopies Are Only for Older Adults."

- **Myth**: Many see colonoscopy as a test strictly for seniors.
- **Fact**: Current guidelines often start screening at **age 45** for average-risk individuals, and **earlier** if family history or personal risk factors exist (IBD, genetic syndromes). Younger adults, especially if symptomatic (rectal bleeding, unexplained weight loss), may need evaluation too.
- **Takeaway**: Colorectal cancer can appear in younger demographics, so ignoring symptoms or skipping screening isn't advisable.

14.2 Common Q&A

14.2.1 "Does Removing the Gallbladder Affect Digestion?"

- **Answer**: The **gallbladder** stores and concentrates **bile** but doesn't produce it; your liver still makes bile continuously. Post-cholecystectomy, bile drips directly into the intestine, sometimes leading to mild diarrhea or bloating initially. Most adapt well, with minimal long-term issues.

- **Practical Note**: A small subset may develop "post-cholecystectomy syndrome," needing dietary tweaks (low-fat meals, or bile-binding agents if diarrhea persists).

14.2.2 "Should I Always Use PPIs for Heartburn?"

- **Answer**: Proton pump inhibitors (PPIs) effectively reduce acid and help heal erosive esophagitis or peptic ulcers, but **long-term** high-dose use has potential downsides (increased risk of bone loss, possible infections, altered gut flora).

- **Recommendation**: If you have mild GERD, try **lifestyle changes** first (weight loss, dietary adjustments, elevating head of bed). Use **short courses** of PPIs or H2 blockers, unless chronic severe disease demands maintenance therapy. Consult your doctor for the proper approach.

14.2.3 "Is Heartburn Always GERD?"

- **Answer**: Not necessarily. **Heartburn** can be due to acid reflux, but also occurs in **functional** chest pain or even from gallbladder disease radiating discomfort to the epigastrium.
- **Practical Note**: Persistent heartburn or regurgitation typically suggests GERD, yet further evaluation is warranted if standard acid suppression fails or alarm features emerge.

14.2.4 "Do I Need a Second Opinion or Specialist Referral?"

- **Answer**: If you're uncertain about a diagnosis, facing major surgery, or your symptoms persist/ worsen despite treatment, a second opinion is wise. For complex GI disorders (advanced IBD, cirrhosis, suspected rare conditions), a **gastroenterologist** or specialized center can provide valuable insights.
- **Practical Note**: Keep all test results, imaging, and pathology reports accessible to streamline the second-opinion process.

14.3 Practical Advice

14.3.1 Medication Adherence & Communication

Adhering to your prescribed plan ensures optimal outcomes—skipped antibiotics or sporadic acid blockers reduce effectiveness, possibly leading to recurrent infections or persistent ulcers. Clear communication with your doctor about side effects or challenges is essential for adjusting therapy promptly.

14.3.2 Dietary Journaling

1. **Identify Triggers**
   - For IBS or reflux, track meals, symptoms, stool patterns. Patterns can reveal lactose intolerance, FODMAP triggers, or acid- exacerbating foods.
2. **Data Sharing**
   - A well-kept journal helps healthcare providers tailor dietary or medication recommendations.

14.3.3 Patient Support Groups & Online Resources

- **Peer Support**
  - Chronic GI issues (Crohn's, celiac) can be isolating; connecting with others fosters emotional well-being and real-world tips.
- **Reputable Web Sources**
  - Gastroenterology societies (AGA, ACG) or celiac/IBD foundations often share guidelines, patient-friendly educational materials.

14.3.4 Stress & Psychological Therapies

GI symptoms frequently intertwine with **stress** or mood. Some practical measures:

- **Relaxation Techniques**: Deep breathing, yoga, mindfulness.
- **Cognitive Behavioral Therapy (CBT)**: Proven beneficial in functional GI complaints and IBS.
- **Counseling**: Family therapy or individual sessions if chronic illness strains personal relationships or mental health.

14.4 Key Terms Recap

- **Spicy Foods vs. Ulcers**: Spices may irritate existing ulcers but aren't primary culprits in ulcer formation (H. pylori, NSAIDs are).
- **Celiac**: True autoimmune disease, not a fad diet; requires gluten-free lifestyle if positive diagnosis.
- **IBS**: A functional disorder lacking endoscopic findings, diagnosed via Rome IV criteria.
- **Gallbladder Removal**: Typically doesn't severely impair digestion; liver continually produces bile.

- **PPIs**: Acid-suppressive medications used judiciously, short-term unless chronic GERD or serious conditions require prolonged usage.

14.5 Quick Quiz

1. **Multiple Choice**: Which statement is **incorrect** regarding celiac disease?

   a) It's an autoimmune reaction to gluten in wheat, barley, rye.

   b) It can cause villous atrophy and malabsorption.

   c) It's a fabricated dietary trend with no actual autoimmune basis.

   d) Adherence to a strict gluten-free diet leads to symptom improvement.

2. **True or False**: A normal colonoscopy means you cannot have IBS.

3. **Fill in the Blank**: If you frequently experience unexplained GI symptoms, it can be helpful to keep a _____ to identify potential dietary triggers and symptom patterns.

4. **Which complication is most concerning with prolonged, high-dose PPI use if not monitored?**

   a) Iron overload

   b) Increased risk of Clostridioides difficile infection

c) Reduced sugar tolerance

d) Kidney stone formation

5. **Short Answer**: Name one reason why a second opinion can be beneficial if you're scheduled for major GI surgery (e.g., colectomy or Whipple procedure).

Answers

1. **(c) It's a fabricated dietary trend with no actual autoimmune basis** – This is false. Celiac disease is a legitimate autoimmune disorder.

2. **False** – IBS can occur despite normal endoscopy, being a functional problem.

3. **Food (Dietary) Journal** – A record of what you eat, symptom timings, and severity.

4. **(b) Increased risk of Clostridioides difficile infection** – Prolonged PPI use can alter gut flora, raising C. diff risk, among other side effects.

5. **Example**: "A second opinion ensures you explore all medical or less invasive options, verify the necessity of surgery, or discuss advanced techniques that might improve outcomes."

Concluding Note

Dispelling **misconceptions** about digestive health—from "spicy foods cause ulcers" to whether IBS is "all in your head"—allows individuals and families to make **well-informed decisions** about their GI care. **Colonoscopy** isn't just for older adults; **celiac disease** is indeed real, and a normal scope doesn't exclude **IBS**. Continual communication with healthcare professionals, medication adherence, and supportive lifestyle measures remain the cornerstone of effective GI management.

By combining the knowledge gained throughout these chapters with self-advocacy—like **seeking second opinions** or joining support groups—you can better navigate the complexities of gastrointestinal well-being.

Chapter 15: Glossary & Additional Resources

15.1 Glossary of GI Terms

Below is an **alphabetical** selection of **key gastroenterological terms** introduced throughout the book. Each term includes a concise definition to aid quick recall or further study.

Achalasia
A motility disorder where the lower esophageal sphincter (LES) fails to relax properly, causing difficulty swallowing and food stasis in the esophagus.

Acid Reflux
Backflow of stomach acid into the esophagus due to LES weakness or inappropriate relaxation, contributing to GERD symptoms (heartburn, regurgitation).

Adenomatous Polyp
A precancerous lesion in the colon that can progress to carcinoma if untreated; includes tubular, tubulovillous, and villous subtypes.

Ascites

Accumulation of fluid in the peritoneal cavity, commonly seen in cirrhosis and portal hypertension.

Barrett's Esophagus

A precancerous condition where chronic GERD transforms the normal squamous epithelium in the distal esophagus into columnar epithelium, elevating esophageal adenocarcinoma risk.

Bile

A liver-produced fluid stored in the gallbladder, essential for emulsifying and absorbing dietary fats.

Biologics (Anti-TNF, etc.)

Advanced immunomodulatory medications used in moderate-severe IBD or autoimmune hepatitis to control inflammation by targeting specific cytokines or cell adhesion molecules.

Brush Border

The microvilli-laden surface of small intestinal enterocytes, carrying enzymes (lactase, sucrase) crucial for nutrient breakdown and absorption.

Celiac Disease
An autoimmune disorder triggered by dietary gluten (wheat, barley, rye) causing villous atrophy, leading to malabsorption and various systemic effects.

Cholecystitis
Inflammation of the gallbladder, typically due to a stone obstructing the cystic duct. Presents with RUQ pain, fever, leukocytosis.

Chronic Pancreatitis
Progressive inflammatory damage to the pancreas resulting in exocrine and endocrine insufficiency (steatorrhea, diabetes), often from alcohol or genetic causes.

Cirrhosis
End-stage liver scarring that disrupts normal architecture, leading to portal hypertension and complications (varices, ascites, encephalopathy).

Colonoscopy
Endoscopic exam of the colon (and sometimes terminal ileum), crucial for polyp detection/removal and colon cancer screening.

Crohn's Disease

A type of IBD marked by transmural inflammation and skip lesions, potentially affecting any GI segment from mouth to anus.

Diverticulosis

Presence of small outpouchings (diverticula) in the colon wall, often asymptomatic but can bleed or become inflamed (diverticulitis).

Encopresis

Fecal soiling from chronic stool withholding and overflow in children, typically due to functional constipation.

Endoscopy

General term for minimally invasive scope procedures (EGD, colonoscopy, sigmoidoscopy) allowing direct visualization and biopsy of GI mucosa.

ERCP (Endoscopic Retrograde Cholangiopancreatography)

Combined endoscopy and fluoroscopy to diagnose or treat biliary/pancreatic duct issues, removing stones or placing stents.

Esophageal pH Monitoring

A 24-hour test measuring acid reflux severity, aiding GERD diagnosis when clinical findings are uncertain.

Fecal Calprotectin

A stool marker indicating bowel inflammation, helping differentiate IBD from IBS or functional disorders.

FODMAPs

Fermentable carbs (fructans, galactans, lactose, etc.) that can aggravate IBS symptoms by increasing gas and fluid in the intestines.

GERD

Gastroesophageal reflux disease; acid reflux causing esophagitis, heartburn, possibly leading to Barrett's if chronic and severe.

H. pylori

Helicobacter pylori, a stomach bacterium causing chronic gastritis, peptic ulcers, and sometimes gastric cancer or MALT lymphoma.

IBS

Irritable bowel syndrome; a functional GI disorder characterized by abdominal pain, altered bowel habits (IBS-D, IBS-C, IBS-M), and normal imaging/labs.

Inflammatory Bowel Disease (IBD)
Chronic inflammatory GI tract disorders (Crohn's disease, ulcerative colitis), distinct from IBS by visible inflammation on endoscopy and histology.

Malabsorption
Impaired nutrient absorption resulting from villous damage (celiac), enzyme deficits (chronic pancreatitis), or short bowel.

NAFLD/NASH
Non-alcoholic fatty liver disease (NAFLD) or steatohepatitis (NASH) from metabolic syndrome, can progress to cirrhosis.

NSAIDs
Nonsteroidal anti-inflammatory drugs that can cause peptic ulcers or exacerbate IBD if used long-term without prophylaxis.

Pancreatic Enzyme Replacement
Pancrelipase supplements assisting digestion in exocrine insufficiency (chronic pancreatitis, post-surgery).

Portal Hypertension

Elevated portal venous pressure in cirrhosis or portal vein obstruction, leading to varices, splenomegaly, ascites.

PPIs (Proton Pump Inhibitors)

Medications (e.g., omeprazole) suppressing stomach acid production, healing GERD, ulcers, or erosive gastritis.

Rome IV Criteria

Diagnostic guidelines for functional GI disorders like IBS, focusing on symptom patterns and absence of alarm features.

Transmural Inflammation

Involvement of the entire thickness of the bowel wall, characteristic of Crohn's disease lesions.

Zollinger-Ellison Syndrome

Gastrin-secreting tumor (gastrinoma) causing excessive acid production, recurrent or severe peptic ulcers.

15.3 Additional Resources & References

15.3.1 Reputable Websites for GI Information

1. **American College of Gastroenterology (ACG)**
   - www.gi.org
   - Guidelines on screening, patient education tools, "Find a GI" resources.

2. **American Gastroenterological Association (AGA)**
   - www.gastro.org
   - Professional guidelines, patient brochures on various GI disorders.

3. **Centers for Disease Control and Prevention (CDC)**
   - www.cdc.gov
   - Travel advisories, vaccine recommendations, food safety guidelines, outbreak info (e.g., Salmonella, E. coli).

4. **National Institute of Diabetes and Digestive and Kidney Diseases (NIDDK)**
   - www.niddk.nih.gov
   - Detailed resources on diabetes, obesity, liver disease, kidney issues, plus research updates.

5. **Celiac Disease Foundation**
   - www.celiac.org
   - Comprehensive guides to gluten-free living, new research, recipes.

15.3.2 Patient Advocacy & Support Groups

1. **Crohn's & Colitis Foundation**
   - www.crohnscolitisfoundation.org
   - Support groups, events, IBD education, fundraising for research.
2. **IBS Network (UK)** or local IBS societies
   - Self-help info, diet tips, symptom diaries, mental health support.
3. **Hepatitis B Foundation & American Liver Foundation**
   - Educational materials on viral hepatitis, cirrhosis management, transplant support.
4. **Gluten Intolerance Group (GIG)**
   - www.gluten.org
   - Guidance for celiac and gluten sensitivity, local chapters for dietary assistance.

15.3.3 Hotlines & Helplines

- **National Suicide Prevention Lifeline** (U.S.): **988**
  - Chronic GI illness can impact mental health; immediate crisis support.
- **Quit Smoking Hotlines**
  - "1-800-QUIT-NOW" (U.S.). Smoking cessation reduces risk of peptic ulcers, Crohn's flare-ups, and various cancers.

15.3.4 Recommended Reading & Journals

1. **Gastroenterology** (by AGA)
   - A leading peer-reviewed journal on GI research, clinical studies, and reviews.
2. **American Journal of Gastroenterology**
   - Published by ACG, featuring cutting-edge clinical guidelines and trials.
3. **The Gut**
   - British-based journal offering broad coverage of GI research, including functional bowel disorders and endoscopy innovations.
4. **Consumer-Focused Books**
   - Guides by known GI specialists or dietitians offering recipes, lifestyle tips for IBS, IBD, celiac disease, or reflux management.

About the Author

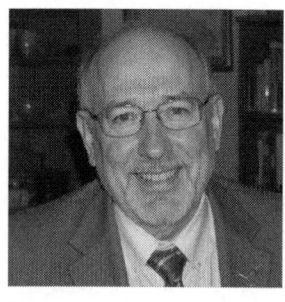 **Richard J. Brooks** is a dedicated medical writer and educator with a lifelong passion for making complex health topics **accessible** to wide audiences. Inspired by the patients, caregivers, and healthcare professionals he's encountered, Richard has spent over two decades

demystifying medical jargon. In addition to his work on the "Medical Terms Made Clear" series, he has contributed to patient guides, clinical review articles, and continuing education materials for health professionals.

Other Books by the Author:

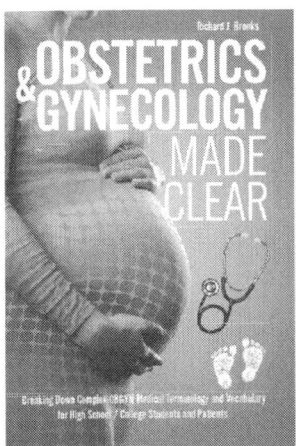 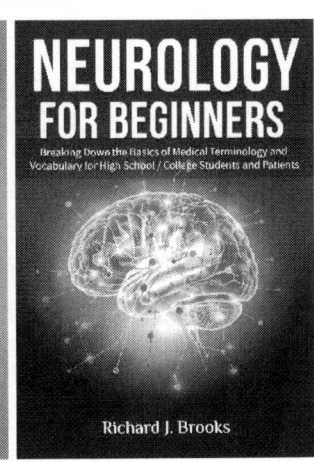

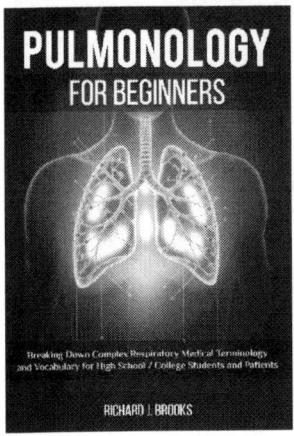

Printed in Dunstable, United Kingdom